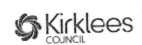

The Magnificent Spilsbury and the Case of the Brides in the Bath

Also by Jane Robins

Rebel Queen

The Magnificent Spilsbury and the Case of the Brides in the Bath

JANE ROBINS

JOHN MURRAY

First published in Great Britain in 2010 by John Murray (Publishers)
An Hachette UK Company

1

© Jane Robins 2010

A CIP catalogue record for this title is available from the British Library

Hardback ISBN 978-1-84854-107-8
Trade paperback ISBN 978-1-84854-108-5

Typeset in 12.25/15 Monotype Bembo by Servis Filmsetting Ltd, Stockport, Cheshire

Printed and bound by Clays Ltd, St Ives plc

John Murray policy is to use papers that are natural, renewable and recyclable products and made from wood grown in sustainable forests. The logging and manufacturing processes are expected to conform to the environmental regulations of the country of origin.

John Murray (Publishers)
338 Euston Road
London NW1 3BH

www.johnmurray.co.uk

For Tom

Contents

I

Bessie

IN THE SUMMER of 1910 the fortunes of Bessie Mundy changed
forever when she decided to take a walk in the pretty Georgian
streets of the Clifton-on-the-Hill district of Bristol. Bessie was a
plain but well-turned-out young woman who was quite alone in
the world. Of course, she had dreamed of meeting a man, settling
down and having a family. But, so far in her life, no Prince
Charming had been sufficiently attracted by her quiet, subservient
manner to whisk her away and make her his wife.

Now, at 33, she was an old maid. It was a humiliating state of
affairs. The passing of too many uneventful years had left Bessie
an almost invisible person, and her chances of deliverance from
the miserable status of spinster had become slim. Had she been
prettier or more vivacious, then her fate might have been different. But the gods seemed to be punishing her for being ordinary
– for possessing a humble, unquestioning nature. It was unfair.
She had the qualities that men were supposed to want in a spouse,
but didn't seem, in practice, to find very alluring.

Nothing about Bessie was actually unattractive. Her dark eyes
were a little vacant, and her face not particularly animated, but
her features were symmetrical and well-proportioned. A surviving photograph suggests that she made the effort to present
herself well, scooping up her abundant frizzy hair under a fashionably wide-brimmed straw hat and dressing neatly in a simple
white blouse and long, plain skirt. But no amount of making the
best of herself could disguise the fact that she had become one of

the unfortunate 'surplus women' who were attracting debate in the press. The country, according to the most excitable commentators, was practically awash with girls who couldn't find a partner at dances.

The predicament stemmed from the tendency for more boys than girls to die in infancy, and was exacerbated by the large numbers of young men who were emigrating to the Colonies. By 1910, British women outnumbered their menfolk by more than half a million, and a sense of panic had crept into the marriage market. According to the popular magazines, a woman should be engaged by the age of 23. At 27 she would be justified in feeling desperate about her marriage prospects. At 30, it might be best to give up hope.

A young, wealthy, beautiful woman would, of course, always find a husband. But the relative lack of power of women in general infuses the pages of the *Matrimonial Times* of 1910. Men seeking women to marry asked for someone young, good-looking, affectionate, domesticated – and with some money too. This last condition was tough in a world where men had the good jobs and women workers were likely to be domestic servants, shop assistants or low-paid factory girls. At least, though, the men who advertised were honest about their requirements.

'Young gentleman', wrote one bachelor, 'good-tempered and affectionate, age 27, height 5 ft 8 in, medium colour, fairly good-looking with own business making about £150 per annum, desires to marry a young Lady, age 25 or less, domesticated and quiet tastes, with about the same income or equivalent capital.' 'Genuine', announced another, 'young Welsh Gentleman, partner in a large drapery establishment, desires to correspond with a religious Lady. Advertiser does not wish to marry her for her money, but would like her to have £1,500 a year in case anything was to happen.'

The women who advertised made the most of any financial incentives they could offer: 'Young orphan, 22, with £450 in cash. I am said to be very pretty, and have never walked out with a man, but want to do so, as I feel very lonely and want to marry a true gentleman, one in regular work who does not drink and gamble on racehorses, but would be willing to buy a nice, comfortable home with my money. I should like my husband to be tall and steady.' Another advertiser took a more forthright tone: 'A domestic, 29 . . . rather stout, with £180 in cash, a good cook and thoroughly domesticated, and quite capable of making any genuine hard-working man a first-rate wife; no use for any flash, fast young men.'

The editor of the paper confessed that there were far more women than men in need of his services. He had, he wrote, 'hundreds of lady clients' on his books, apart from the current advertisers.

So, in the circumstances, it was a great surprise when Bessie, while out walking in Clifton, fell into conversation with a complete stranger who was single and plainly a marriage prospect. Henry Williams was a smooth-talking Londoner, who dressed like a dandy and boasted of being a professional man, making his living by restoring old paintings. There was something out of the ordinary about him – the flamboyance of his clothes, the fact that he appeared to be widely travelled, and an intensity of manner. He was slightly older than Bessie and, in his way, not bad-looking. His physique was good – slim and muscular, as though he were accustomed to physical work, or had spent time in the army. His thin, angular face was presentable enough, but his eyes were slightly unnerving. People described them as penetrating and hypnotic. We do not know whether Bessie's heart raced at the sight of Henry, or if she instantly saw him in a romantic light. But it is clear that she liked him enough, or was sufficiently desperate, to agree to meet him again.

Bessie, at this point in her life, was living in rented rooms, and was away from her family. But her isolation was a relatively recent state of affairs. Until 1904 she had lived in the west country with her father, George Bailey Mundy, a bank manager for the Wiltshire and Dorset Banking Company in Warminster. Her father's two brothers lived nearby – Uncle Frank was a bank manager in Wootton Bassett, and Uncle Herbert an auctioneer and estate agent in Trowbridge. Bessie had an older brother, Howard, but her mother had died when her daughter was only a few weeks old. So George Mundy had raised the two children by himself.

In 1901 George made a will in which he divided his estate between the two children. Howard was to receive most of the household furniture, and Bessie her mother's writing desk, which was kept in the drawing-room of the family home, and her jewellery. A few years later, George became seriously ill, and he died on 11 December 1904. Henry Williams would later claim that Bessie's father had died 'raving mad'.

Bessie's brother Howard and uncles Frank and Herbert now discussed her financial affairs. She had inherited £2,500 – a very considerable sum. But she was, the men decided, 'not a good businesswoman', and would be hopeless at making investments. (Indeed, it was a common belief that 'irresponsibility about money, which is one of the vital affairs in life, is a grave defect in all women'.) So they decided to do the job for her, setting up a trust. Uncle Herbert took the lead, managing the money and ensuring that Bessie received an income of £8 a month for the rest of her life. This would be enough for her to live on – to rent a room, and to buy clothes and food. So Bessie was financially secure, but, for some reason, she now lost contact with her immediate family – moving from place to place as a paying guest, and rarely seeing her brother or uncles. Evidence of her exact whereabouts in the years after her father's death is sketchy, but it seems that she spent eighteen months or two years staying with the Reverend Westlake at the rectory in Sutton Benger, a village in the Wiltshire countryside. Then, at some point, she decided that the town might suit her better, and moved to Bristol.

The city was lively and busy, with plenty to offer a single woman in need of distraction. The big new department stores were stocked with the latest fashions, and the local papers carried advertisements declaring that buyers had returned from Paris and Vienna with 'the very latest and newest productions'. All the talk in 1910 was of the absurd narrowness of ladies' skirts and the monstrous size of their hats. 'Soon an Act of Parliament will be needed to restrict the size of headgear', wrote an anonymous correspondent in the *Bristol Times and Mirror*. The hats, she thought, 'positively extinguished' moderately tall women, 'while the petite individual closely resembles an enormous mushroom on a stalk'.

Bristol also offered the prospect of work. This was the age of female emancipation and the development of careers for women who had failed to find husbands. The papers were full of articles about unmarried girls from modest backgrounds who were entering the workplace in jobs that were – it was to be hoped – more fulfilling than the heart-sinking drudgery of domestic service. Clerical and secretarial work was available, along with shop work, and catering work. 'Marriage, or the cloisters of a Convent or of an old maid's abode, are not now the sole alternatives open to women', observed a writer in Clifton's free newspaper. '"Careers" which in the past were only allowed to men, actresses and adventuresses, now honourably tempt young girls of every situation in life.' The modern girl was apparently no longer fixated on young men; rather she had enlarged her topics of conversations to 'hockey, golf, books . . . and philanthropy'.

And some girls were turning political. The suffragette movement was particularly active in Bristol, where Annie Kenney, the devotee of Christabel Pankhurst, was recruiting and training young women. Her charges, she wrote: 'were wonderful workers; they worked night and day. I had not one voluntary worker, I had scores. I trained speaker after speaker.' In 1909, while Bessie was living in Bristol and those suffragettes in prison were on hunger-strike, some of Annie Kenney's trainees smashed the windows of the city's government buildings, and one – Theresa Garnett – caused national outrage when she shouted 'take that you brute!' at Winston Churchill, as she hit him across the face with a horsewhip at Bristol Temple Meads station and 'knocked his hat about'. In 1910 Mrs Emmeline Pankhurst herself appeared at Bristol's Palace Theatre to argue that the movement had broken down all class distinctions. While titled women were busy chalking the announcement of suffragettes' meetings on the pavements, she proclaimed, a woman of the leisured class and a shoemaker's wife might join together to take out a barrel-organ to raise funds. This was not entirely accurate. The suffragettes attracted more upper-class and educated women than simple girls from ordinary backgrounds.

Bessie, though, was not a particularly active type and not much affected by the lively goings-on in Bristol. Of all the advertisements and reports in local newspapers that give a flavour of life while she was there, there is only one message that stands out as being of particular relevance to her – the offer of 'artificial teeth' that might be purchased for one guinea a set, 'consultations and advice free'. We know that Bessie had decided to have all her teeth pulled out, and replaced by a full set of dentures. False teeth were now within the grasp of almost everyone. In earlier times they had been available only to the rich, and were made of ivory, hippopotamus teeth or – most famously – of the looted teeth of soldiers who died at Waterloo. But new technology led to fake teeth being set in more comfortable, durable vulcanized rubber.

When the patent ran out in 1881, vulcanized rubber dentures became extremely cheap, and poorer people no longer had to live with the pain of rotting teeth. Now, with the help of new anaesthetics, they could have a whole mouthful extracted and a set of dentures instead. False teeth were an aspirational beauty product – as was endlessly illustrated in advertisements showing 'before' and 'after' pictures of young women. 'Look at the illustrations of [the] lady's face above,' said the newspaper advertisement for 'Williams Teeth'. 'One shows the disfiguring effects of missing teeth. The other shows how perfect teeth beautify.' In December 1906 the *Daily Mirror* estimated that 'no fewer than 250,000 teeth have been drawn in London this month'.

In having all her teeth out, Bessie was simply following the fashion. There was nothing extreme, or even unusual, in her action. But in 1910 she did decide upon an action that *was* radical – indeed it was rebellious. That summer, she allowed the Londoner Henry Williams to persuade her to leave the rented rooms that she called home, and to run away with him – an act that threw all the normal rules of courtship to the wind. She spent no time at all to get to know him, and didn't take him to the country to meet Uncle Frank, Uncle Herbert or her brother Howard. In fact, she seems to have told nobody at all about him, and instead allowed herself to be caught up in a heady, whirlwind romance.

For Bessie, to be married was everything. And, as it turned out, she was at this moment particularly anxious for her life to change. She hated her rented rooms. The landlady's husband, Mr Notely, 'certainly did drink . . . and is atrocious at times'. He 'swears and curses', she wrote in a letter, and 'pulls his wife about when he is like this'. Most disturbingly, though, he had on one occasion 'touched' Bessie. She told Henry about the ghastliness of the Notely household, and he responded by telling her to stick with him, and promising her 'a much better life'.

Leaving behind unpaid bills of about £20, and taking nothing with her except a hatbox, Bessie now joined Henry on a journey – probably by train, since he regularly travelled by rail – to the Dorset seaside town of Weymouth. There was something about

Henry that suggested recklessness and abandon, and this awakened in Bessie a desire for excitement and escape.

The couple's choice of a seaside resort made sense. There they could be anonymous, could disappear into the crowds of holiday-makers and day-trippers – and they could be publicly affectionate without attracting undue attention. At the seaside, to be from out-of-town was normal, to be excessively romantic was almost expected, and to flout the normal rules of respectability was pleasurably daring. The *Bristol Times* that summer carried advertisements promoting Weymouth as the 'sunniest and healthiest spot in England . . . the English Naples – the place to spend the holidays'. The town's attractions included 'boating, daily concerts, skating-rinks, steamboat excursions, coaching trips, Pavilion and Theatre', an impressive pier, and a particularly pleasing promenade that was two miles long.

In truth, Weymouth is probably the most sedate of the seaside towns in the story that follows. It had not succumbed to the greatest excesses of the national enthusiasm for holiday entertainments, but had kept hold of the dignity that the Georgian age had conferred on it. George III's visits to Weymouth had made it famous, and the buildings along the front retained a Georgian elegance. The streets behind, though, were modern, and Bessie and Henry, when they arrived, chose to look for lodgings in Rodwell Avenue, a pleasantly curved road of solid Edwardian houses, five minutes' walk from the harbour.

Mrs Maud Crabb and her husband Fred lived at no. 14, and rented out rooms. Maud later remembered that on 22 August 1910 a man and a woman called at the house. The man had asked 'Do you let apartments?' and when Maud said yes, he requested a sitting-room and two bedrooms. Maud was struck by the couple's lack of luggage: he had only a small bag and she a hat-box.

'He told me his name was Williams,' said Maud, 'but did not say who the woman was. On the Wednesday evening, 24 August, after they had been here two days I asked the woman how I should address her. She said, "I am Miss Mundy." He said, "It won't be that much longer, we intend to be married."'

The wedding, said Henry, was to take place in a few days time – and he asked Maud and Fred Crabb to be witnesses. Fred said that he was a working man, and he would lose half a day's work if he came along. Henry replied, 'That will be all right. I will pay you for any loss of time.' So the Crabbs agreed, and on 26 August, the little group of bride, groom, landlady and her husband walked together from 14 Rodwell Avenue to the Weymouth register office. There were no other guests, and the witnesses had known the bride and groom just four days.

It is to be hoped that Bessie was happy on the day of her odd little wedding. Within a short period of time, however, it became clear to Maud Crabb that all was not well. Henry Williams, she said, 'would never let me speak to his wife alone, if he could possibly help it. She always seemed afraid of him, and seemed incapable of opposing anything that he said.' And there was a problem with money. When Fred asked Henry to pay for his loss of income, Henry prevaricated and promised to pay at a later date. But the days slipped by, and no money was produced. And by 13 September, the payments for the Williams' board and lodging were two weeks behind.

From Bessie's point of view, money became the dominating feature of her marriage. On the day of her wedding, undoubtedly at Henry's insistence, she wrote to her family's solicitor asking for a copy of her father's will, which duly arrived in Weymouth a few days later. And during the first week of the marriage both she and Henry wrote to Uncle Herbert, telling him about the wedding, and asking for money.

'We cannot say at present how long we shall remain in Weymouth', wrote Henry on 29 August. 'Bessie hopes you will forward as much money as possible at your earliest (by registered letter). Am pleased to say Bessie is in perfect health, and both are looking forward to a bright and happy future.' A postscript signed 'Bessie Williams' reads simply – 'With my kind regards, I am very happy indeed.' Two days later, Bessie also wrote to Uncle Herbert, thanking him for a money order of £10, but explaining that she and Henry had 'promised each other faithfully to throw in our lot together, which is only natural', and so needed a lot more cash. 'My husband and myself have made up our minds to set up a house and commence business', she wrote. 'My husband is a first-class picture restorer, so now you know our programme. I therefore trust that you will forward money at your earliest . . .'

On 2 September, a week after the wedding, Henry took Bessie to see Arthur Eaton, a solicitor with offices on the Esplanade in Weymouth. Arthur hadn't met Henry before, and asked him where he came from, but Henry evaded the question. At the meeting, said Arthur, Henry 'did practically all the talking. The woman simply acquiesced when anything was put to her by me.' Bessie, Henry said, was due a good deal of money under her father's will. At the very least, she was owed back payments of about £123, and she wished to receive this money without further delay.

At home in Trowbridge, Uncle Herbert was suspicious. It had been bad enough that the first he knew of Bessie's new husband was a postcard from her, written on her wedding day, stating simply: 'Dear Uncle, I have got married today, my husband is writing to you tonight', and signed, with puzzling formality, 'B. Williams'. But to have this terse communication quickly followed by a succession of requests for cash was, at the very least, unsettling. Uncle Herbert later said, 'I put every obstacle in the way, and instructed my solicitor to delay matters as much as possible.' But consultations between Uncle Herbert and his solicitor resulted in the depressing conclusion that, legally, nothing could be done to prevent the surrender of £138 that was due to Bessie in interest payments that had accrued on her investments.

Thankfully, the capital sum of £2,500 was safe and could be kept in the trust.

Early in the morning of 13 September 1910 Henry Williams asked his landlady, Maud Crabb, 'Has the postman been?'

'He has gone,' Maud replied, 'but there is nothing for you.'

'My wife is expecting a cheque,' said Henry. 'I've got nothing, it's my wife who's got it all.'

And a cheque for more than £100 did arrive that day, at Arthur Eaton's office in Weymouth. At 9 a.m. Henry took Bessie to see the solicitor, and asked, 'Can you let us have cash for it?' Arthur suggested that the couple wait for the cheque to be cleared, but Henry was insistent. He really wanted cash, and he wanted it immediately. Arthur relented, and sent the cheque to be cashed at the bank. While they were waiting for the money, Henry asked whether the amount could be collected in gold rather than cash. But cash it was. Arthur, in Henry's presence, advised Bessie to put the money in the Post Office Savings Bank. 'She said she would,' said Arthur, 'and he signified his approval of this being done. I paid Mrs Williams herself the amount in cash and they left.'

While Bessie and Henry were out, a telegram for Henry arrived at the Crabbs' house in Rodwell Avenue. At 11 a.m. Henry returned, alone. He read the telegram, and told Maud: 'I've got to go to London at once on important business, when my wife comes in tell her if I am not home tonight, I shall be home next Monday.'

'He took his hand-bag and left,' said Maud. As he went, he explained that Bessie's money had come through, and said 'See that she pays you.'

At about one o'clock Bessie returned to Rodwell Avenue, and asked if Henry had come home. 'When I told her he was gone, she was greatly upset,' said Maud. Henry had left behind a post-card for Bessie, on which he had written in pencil: 'I have just received a telegram from the Doctor and have to go to London at once. Shall not be home till tomorrow.'

A letter written by Henry, for Bessie to hand to the Crabbs, suggested that, rather than returning the following day, he might not be home for some time. 'I do not know how long I shall be away', it began, and then suggested that the Crabbs take care of Bessie's 'will settlement' and put it in a secure box. 'I shall give you 10s for your trouble.' He explained that Bessie received £8 a month from her trust, and could pay the Crabbs 30 shillings a month for board and lodging. 'You will find her no trouble', he concluded, 'so I hope you will make her comfortable until my return.'

In addition to the postcard, there was a letter for Bessie:

> Dearest,
> I fear you have blasted all my bright hopes of a happy future. I have caught from you a disease which is called the bad disorder, for you to be in such a state proves you could not have kept yourself morally clean. It reminds of what you told me in ref. to the imorality of Mr Notely. Anyhow you have got the disease somehow. I don't wish to say you have had connections with another man and got it from him. But it is either that or through not keeping yourself clean. Now for the sake of my health and honour and yours too I must go to London and act intirly under the Doctors advice to get proply cured of this disease. It will cost me a great deal of money because it might take years before I am cured . . .

The letter was filled with instructions. She must tell people that he had gone to France on business. Only Uncle Herbert should be told the 'truth' about Henry's disease. And, if Uncle Herbert should ask about the money:

> tell him that you kept all the money which was sent to you in a leather bag and two days after I had gone you happened to go on the beach and fall asleep and when you woke the Bag of money was gone.
> . . . If you do not carry out every word of my advice you will cause a lot of trouble and the whole affair will be in the Police

Court and you will bring disgrace on yourself and relations. Now study this letter and whatever you do stick to everything you say, never alter it or else you will get mixed up and make a fool of yourself. When you have read this letter take it in the street and tear it up.

There was a relentless repetition of the message. 'Now stick to every word of this and never alter it or else serious trouble and disgrace will fall on all . . . now tare this letter up at once and throw the pieces on the road.'

'That same day,' said Maud, 'she was very much distressed and had an hysterical fit which made it necessary for me to call in Dr Miller . . . She was very ill.'

Bessie did have the presence of mind, however, to send a telegram to Uncle Herbert, stating simply: 'Husband left me today taken money, please send me some, writing. Bessie.'

The letter that she sent the next day was an outpouring of misery and remorse.

Uncle, I am very sorry, and know I have worried you, also myself. I was so ill I was told yesterday I had to be carried up to bed by the doctor. I also can't help breaking down. Of course I miss him, but of course I feel on the other hand, it is a mercy I am rid of him . . . I am worrying also, because I feel you are all against me now. I feel I have disgraced you all. The doctor told Mrs Crabb I shall have to shake it off or else I shall not get over it. Dear uncle, do forgive me . . . I do hope my husband will be caught, of course the Police are on [the case], they have issued a warrant. I quite see now what I have fallen into, and feel I have disgraced myself for life.

On the day that Henry absconded with Bessie's money, her brother Howard's wife came to visit, and three days later Howard came himself, and found Bessie still 'very much distressed, and hysterical. She had practically no clothing, and was penniless and in debt to the landlady Mrs Crabb.' In fact, she was in such a terrible state that Howard judged her to be unfit to travel. After a while, though, he took her to his home in nearby Poole, and she spent two or three months there convalescing, and working out how to proceed with her life.

Something persuaded her that her best option was to return to Bristol, and by the early part of 1911 she was back in the city, back in her old life of a single woman in rented rooms, but carrying the extra burden of the shame and humiliation of having run away with a man who had turned out to be, not simply cruel and dishonourable, but a cad and a criminal.

To her credit, though, Bessie now decided to make something of herself, and to acquire some skills that might be useful in the workplace. She enrolled at the Civil Service Institute, a college that offered training courses for prospective soldiers, bankers, accountants, auctioneers, architects, teachers and secretaries. It was the last of these that seemed most suitable, and she joined the bookkeeping, shorthand and typewriting classes run by the principal, James Griffiths. Bessie could expect to double her income on becoming a secretary – a job that was seen as a neat fit with the female character. An essential quality in a secretary, wrote Annie Davis in 1913, was that 'woman's birthright – Tact'. This is the 'inestimable quality' which leads a woman

> to say or do the right thing at the right moment, or which enables her to observe silence, if such a course is the better policy. Tact is at the head of a long train of other admirable qualities, for the tactful woman is invariably considerate for others, courteous, patient, cheerful and ready at all times to give of her best. The possession of Tact will enable a girl to adapt herself to circumstances and surroundings, and will help her to fit easily into any position in which she may be placed.

It was a role that suited Bessie's submissive, compliant character.

Bessie attended the college for nearly a year, and during that time became sufficiently friendly with James Griffiths to tell him the extraordinary story of her relationship with Henry Williams. While in Weymouth, she said, he tried to get from her the full amount of her inheritance – £2,500 – but had been stopped by her solicitors. When the smaller cheque, for the interest, had arrived – he had taken the money from her on the pretext of paying for the furniture that they would need for their future marital home.

But all prospects of a career for Bessie receded when in March 1912, eighteen months after the disaster at Weymouth, she decided to take a fortnight's holiday in the nearby seaside town of Weston-super-Mare. There is no record of why she wanted to go to the resort out of season, when it would undoubtedly be cold and a trifle bleak. But we know that she *did* go, and that she rented a room from an acquaintance of the family, Sarah Tuckett. We also know that one day, while walking along the promenade, she once again ran into Henry Williams. And, with astonishing alacrity, she again fell under his spell. Instead of going straight to the police and having him arrested, she was quickly persuaded that he loved her and intended to be a loving, caring husband. As her brother Howard said later, she 'was always a woman who would be easily led.'

Henry explained that he had been trying to find her for some time, that the business with a 'disease' had all been a terrible mistake, and that he now wanted to make amends and provide her with 'a settled comfortable home'. We know the line he took in persuading Bessie, because he set it down in a number of letters. He wanted, he told Mrs Tuckett, 'to prove myself not only a true husband but a gentleman and finally make my peace step by step with all those who have been kind to Bessie'. He also wrote to Bessie's brother, Howard – employing ridiculously archaic language:

> I know not how I shall offend in dedicating my unpolished lines to you . . . Let the past sink into oblivion. I account myself

highly honoured, and vow to take advantage of every future day that the great powers have ordained untill the miserable past is absolutely outlived and a character established which will be worthy of your appreciation . . . No husband could possibly be more sorry than myself for what has occurred.

A letter to Uncle Herbert was similarly filled with contrition. Henry vowed 'to take advantage of every hour and day for the future that Bessie and I are spared to outlive the past and to prove myself before the eyes of my wife and her relatives a true and worthy husband'.

His words rang hollow, not least because they were accompanied by a chilling undercurrent of menace. Bessie's relatives and Mrs Tuckett were plainly concerned for her – but Henry warned them off. It would be 'dangerous to try and do us harm or endeavour to make our lives miserable', he wrote. 'It appears that many people would rather stir up strife than try and make peace . . . why in the name of Heaven and Christianity do people like to constantly interfere and stir up past trouble . . . Life after all is not finished yet.'

Bessie, too, wrote letters about her sudden change in circumstances. She implored her brother Howard to 'try and forgive and forget the past, as I have done . . . I know my husband better now than ever before . . . you will be pleased to know I am perfectly happy.' And, when Uncle Herbert failed to respond to a letter from Henry, she wrote to him:

> My dear Uncle,
> I am writing this letter quite unknown to my husband, and according to my own conscience. I am deeply moved for not receiving a line from you. I must admit that I know my husband now better than ever I did. I also have every reason to believe that he intends to redeem the past, and a happy future is before me. But I really must point out that to stir up the past would not only make us somewhat miserable, but worse of all if my husband were to leave me again through any of my relatives

interferences, my life would not be worth living, I should never get over it . . . it is impossible to injure my husband, who I love, without injuring me. For my sake, forget and forgive, and do let me have a line from you,

    Yrs, with love,

    Bessie

The letter, written in Henry's distinctive style, suggests a picture of him at his wife's side, dictating as she obediently writes.

When she had first met Henry in 1910, Bessie very soon found herself at his side, in a solicitor's office, talking about her finances. Now, nearly two years later, the same thing happened. Henry took her along to see Wadsworth Lillington, a solicitor who practised in Weston-super-Mare. He told the lawyer that 'he had contracted a contagious disease quite independently of his wife, and that he left her at Weymouth from a fear of communicating such disease to her'. No mention was made of his atrocious allegations against Bessie, or of the fact that he had robbed her of her money. Instead, Henry said that she had 'advanced' him the sum of £150 for the purpose of 'discharging certain debts'. When asked directly by Mr Lillington whether this was the case, Bessie replied that yes, it was as her husband had stated. Mr Lillington suggested that Henry give his wife a promissory note for £150, and he agreed to do so – and the solicitor agreed to send a letter to Uncle Herbert, informing him of this transaction, and of Henry's commitment to his marriage.

Uncle Herbert, nonetheless, continued to think of Henry as a thoroughly bad lot, unlike Bessie who accepted her husband's protestations of remorse. It is impossible to say whether she was charmed by him, in love with him or simply weak and gullible – but she once again surrendered her will to his, and went away to live with him. That March they took rooms in Woolwich, a town to the south-east of London. But they did not stay there long. In April, the couple went to Ramsgate on the Kent coast, and from there Bessie wrote to Uncle Herbert saying that she had 'thoroughly tested' her husband's affection towards her, and found it to be 'more than satisfactory'. Therefore, she continued, her great desire was that the will and settlement that was the source of her wealth should be made out in her married name. They had not been in Ramsgate long before Henry suggested that they move again, this time to the nearby seaside town of Herne Bay, and set up a proper home together.

It must have seemed to Bessie that her husband had chosen an exciting location for their new life. Herne Bay, on the north Kent coast, was a bustling resort – made popular by the fact that day-trippers from London could visit by Thames steamboat or the train. And that spring the town was particularly busy because of the unseasonably hot weather. On 10 May the temperature rose to 75 degrees in the shade, making winter clothing 'a burden' and tempting many to indulge in a 'refreshing dip from the beach or a bathing machine'. On 18 May the south-east of England was still 'revelling in the most glorious and earliest summer that has ever come before English June entered the calendar'. And, by the time the Whitsun bank holiday arrived at the end of the month, the town was packed with holiday visitors and 'excursionists'.

That weekend boats were out in force on the 'perfectly calm sea', and 'bathers of both sexes were splashing in the waves'. Some people simply spent the day sitting out in the deckchairs in the gardens, or on the grass of the Downs, while the band of the Royal Irish Rifles played. At the Pier Pavilion theatre, the Jollity Boys drew an audience of between 3,000 and 4,000 people. On the beach, 'lovers were spending a day of bliss in the shelter of groynes', while children paddled in the sea or built sandcastles. 'The landaus were in request, and the motor coaches to Canterbury were filled. There was all the animation of the season, all the joy of life and the search of pleasure.'

Herne Bay's three picture palaces had a full programme, each showing at least four films a week, which could be seen for threepence or sixpence. The Paragon on the High Street advertised itself as 'the Original Electric Theatre' to be chosen for films presented with 'Rock steadiness, Maximum Light, Perfect Definition, Without Flicker'. Detective stories, comedies, dramas and westerns were interspersed with newsreels. Fashion news was relayed from Paris; the sports news included the English cricket team arriving from Australia, 'bringing home the Ashes'. But overshadowing all else, were the many heart-wrenching reports in the picture palaces and the newspapers of the sinking of the *Titanic*, and the death of 1,517 of her passengers.

The disaster in a distant ice-packed sea was instantly recognized as a momentous historic event, and lent a chill to the otherwise sun-drenched holiday season of 1912. The Herne Bay press carried an eye-witness account by local woman, Miss Kate Buss, who was among the 706 survivors. Quite by chance, she said, she had heard the call of 'any more ladies on deck? . . . ladies first', and had found a place in a lifeboat, leaving behind male friends who did not wear lifebelts, thinking it unnecessary. 'With such a big ship, and Marconi communication, they thought we would have had relief before she sank.' But of course, there was no relief, and from the lifeboat Kate Buss saw the ship go down, with all her friends on board. 'I cried so much,' she wrote, 'when I knew that we had lost our friends, and it's simply awful to see the distressed widows and distracted parents. No, never as long as I live shall I forget it, nor the brave souls who I know have perished.' The musicians who went down with the ship, 'were such nice men,' she remembered, 'and I hear that they were playing "Nearer my God to Thee".'

In early June there was a brief spell of 'copious showers', and the gardens of Herne Bay that had threatened to become a brown wilderness sprang back to life. At this time, the reports about the *Titanic* began to subside, and with the re-emergence of the sun, pleasure-seeking activities once more dominated local news. Herne Bay's famous roller-skating rink was packed with skaters and ice-dancers, and the town's roller hockey team managed an 11-0 win over neighbouring Margate.

There was now a sudden excess of heat, and the temperature in the shade rose to 80 degrees. Fifty new bathing cabins were opened before a crowd of several hundred people. The band of the First South Wales Borderers played; swimming races were held and, to hearty applause, an expert calling himself Professor Broadhurst gave an exhibition of his swimming and diving skills, his feats including 'imitating a seal and a porpoise, turning somersaults and drinking milk under water'.

Bessie and Henry had turned up in Herne Bay some time that May. Miss Carrie Rapley, who worked in a local estate agent's office, remembered Henry coming to see her on 20 May to enquire about renting a small house. Miss Rapley said that no. 80 High Street was free and could be rented at £18 a year. There was some discussion over whether Henry might be allowed to pay monthly. Carrie Rapley asked what references he could give, and when he replied 'none', she said that, in that case, she couldn't do business with him. Henry then explained that he couldn't give references as he had been living in rented rooms and abroad, adding that 'I might as well tell you my wife is a notch above me, in fact her father was a Bank Manager.' Miss Rapley's boss, Mr Frederic Wilbee, then arrived at the office and joined in the discussion. It was eventually agreed that Henry could rent the house, despite the lack of references, paying monthly with a month's rent in advance.

On the 29 May, Bessie wrote to Uncle Herbert from the house at 80 High Street, describing Herne Bay as 'very select and healthy'. Henry, she said, had already spent £80 on furniture, adding:

> but he does not mind that so long as I am happy. He is a thor-
> ough good husband, and I am happy as any woman breathing,

in fact, everybody seems to take to him, of course he gets rather popular because he is a dealer in works of art, and has had some good strokes of luck. He is not only a good and kind husband, but it is said, and I confirm it, that he is one of the most interesting men that anyone wished to speak to, and a very keen business man also.

She invited Uncle Herbert to visit as a paying guest. But Herbert Mundy remained suspicious of Henry, and decided to keep his distance. He didn't visit, and kept his responses to Bessie's letters to a minimum. When, on 6 June, she wrote to him asking for details of her investments, he duly supplied the list. And when she asked for any outstanding money she was owed to be sent to Herne Bay, he despatched it.

Henry presented himself as a stylish man-about-town, wearing a frock-coat, silk hat and long gold chain as he went about the local streets. He seemed to take great pride in the marital home, removing a broken knocker from the front door and attaching a new one. He fixed a brass plate to the door with 'H. Williams, Art Dealer, Pictures, China, Curios and Antique Furniture bought' engraved upon it. This change from his earlier profession of 'picture restorer', however, did not entail a dramatic alteration in lifestyle. It seems that Bessie never saw him actually do any work, either as a picture restorer or as an antique dealer.

The local journeyman baker, Percy Millgate, lived next door to the couple and delivered their bread. He saw them every day, and formed the impression that, despite Henry's flamboyant personal style, they lived 'very quietly'. Carrie Rapley saw Bessie and Henry once or twice that summer. On one occasion they came to her house, 'Fairy Glen', because, said Henry, his wife wanted to see a clergyman and 'I am told there is one living about here.' Miss Rapley made a recommendation, and Henry instructed her to go to see him alone while he waited for her. In conversation with Miss Rapley he said that he 'dabbled in paints'. 'What do you mean?' she asked. He said, 'My father was a bit of an artist,' and began to talk about Florence. He also invited Miss Rapley to tea at number 80. 'I did not go to their house for tea,' she said later, 'and did not see Mrs Williams again until the 6 July, when she was standing at her front door at about 1 p.m. I did not speak to her on this occasion, although she beckoned me with her hand.'

On 19 June Henry took Bessie along to the office of Phillip de Vere Annersley, a solicitor with offices on the High Street, and instructed the lawyer to prepare wills for each of them. Bessie would leave Henry all her worldly goods, and he in return would bequeath all he had to her. A few days later they returned to Mr de Vere Annersley's office to sign the drafts. On 3 July Bessie visited alone, and gave her approval to her will. Then, on 8 July, she and Henry came back once more, to hear the wills read over. The procedures were now complete, and Henry paid the lawyer's fees that day.

While all this was going on, it seems that Henry decided that there was one element missing in the Williams' life at 80 High Street. The house, he felt, would be much better if it had a bath in it. Some time early in July he visited Adolphus Hill, an iron-monger who had a shop at 46 William Street, a two-minute walk away from 80 High Street. 'I see you have a bath there, what do you want for it?' he asked. Henry was referring to a cast-iron bath, five feet six inches long, and 'the usual depth and breadth'. Mr Hill said that he could have the bath for 'about two pounds'. Henry replied that he would think about it, and left the shop. A day or two later Bessie called in to see the bath, and asked if she could have it for the lower price of £1 17s 6d. 'Mr Williams told me to say,' she said, 'that you must let us have it.' Mr Hill observed that she appeared 'excited and agitated'. Something about her manner disturbed him and he 'let her have it at the price she offered, to get rid of her'. The bath was delivered to 80

High Street the next day, 5 July. No arrangements were made for plumbing it in – so it had to be filled and emptied manually, using buckets.

Five days later, on 10 July, Henry took Bessie to the surgery of Frank French, a newly qualified doctor who had set up a practice in Herne Bay. Henry spoke for Bessie, and explained that she had had a fit the previous day. The doctor asked Bessie if she had any history of fits, and she replied that she had never had any before, but mentioned that her father had 'died demented', though she could not remember what particular illness he had suffered from. Dr French examined her tongue, since epileptics were known to bite their tongues during a fit. But Bessie's tongue appeared to be normal. Nonetheless, he thought epilepsy the most likely diagnosis, and prescribed the appropriate medicine.

On the morning of Friday, 12 July, Henry once more appeared at the home of Dr French, this time alone. His wife, he said, had just had another fit. So Dr French went to 80 High Street, a three-minute walk away, where he found Bessie in bed. 'She was not in a fit then,' he said, 'and I could find no evidence of a fit.' Her hands were 'moist', he noted. But this was the height of the blistering 1912 summer, and the night had been extremely hot. Bessie said she felt 'headachy', which, in the doctor's view, was compatible with the after-effects of an epileptic fit, so he prescribed more medicine. That afternoon, he called again at the house. No one was at home but, said Dr French, 'as I was going out of the gate the husband and wife came up. She still complained of lassitude and headache.'

That day, Bessie wrote to Uncle Herbert.

My dear Uncle,
I am very sorry to say that last Tuesday night I had a very bad fit and again on Thursday, and now I feel very weak and suffer with my nerves and headache. It has evidently shocked my

whole system, my husband has been exceedingly kind to me, and done his utmost for my benefit. He has proved himself as good a husband that any woman could wish to have, besides doing all he can for me, in many ways which I shall never forget, he has procured the attendance of the very best doctors in the town, who are constantly giving me medical treatment, and visiting me day and night. I do not like to bother my relatives with my misfortune, but my husband has strictly advised me to write them all and inform them of my breakdown in health. Previous to my breakdown, I had made out my Will, which was afterwards confirmed by a Solicitor, Counsel and witness, in which I have left everything which I am entitled to at my decease to my husband, which after all is only natural, for I love my husband.

Believe me,

Yrs affectionately,

Bessie Williams

The following morning, said Henry, he and Bessie got up together at 7.30. He went out for a stroll, and to buy some fish. When he returned, at about 8 o'clock, he went into the dining-room and called out to his wife. There was no answer, so he checked the bedroom. She wasn't there, so he looked in the back bedroom, where the bath was. 'She was in the bath,' he said. 'Her head was right under the water, submerged . . . I spoke to her, raised her head. I pulled her head right out of the water and rested it on the side of the bath. I then went straight for Dr French.'

Frank French was at home on the morning of Saturday, 13 July. In fact, at 8 o'clock he was still undressed when his servant brought him a note from Henry Williams, written in pencil, urging him to 'come at once, I am afraid my wife is dead'. He dressed as fast as he could, then accompanied Henry to 80 High Street. There he found Bessie 'in the bath, her head submerged' with her mouth at the level of the water. If he thought it odd that

Henry had left his wife with her head under water, he did not say so. Dr French raised Bessie's head, and felt her pulse, but there was none. So, with Henry's help, he lifted her naked body out of the bathwater, which, he noted, was tepid and three-quarters of the way up the bath. He removed both Bessie's upper and lower sets of false teeth – which were still perfectly in place – and tried desperately to revive her. With Henry holding down his wife's tongue, Dr French kept up his attempts at artificial respiration for more than half an hour. 'A lot of froth came from her mouth,' he said, 'blowing across the floor. She certainly had water in the stomach, because in pressing her stomach, some water ran from her mouth, showing she had swallowed water.' He noted that, although dead, she was still clasping a large bar of soap in her right hand.

There was no sign of a struggle, and Dr French concluded that she had died from drowning following an epileptic fit. True, he had never seen Bessie having a fit and had small ground to go on, and her tongue was not bitten, but, he reflected, she had not disagreed with his diagnosis when he had interviewed her in the presence of her husband. When he examined her body later, he found no evidence of any heart trouble which might explain her collapse in the bath. And he did not suspect foul play. Henry Williams had, he thought, done all he could for his wife. And he seemed greatly upset by her death, sobbing bitterly at certain times in the following days. When asked by the local coroner, Rutley Mowll, Dr French said that he thought there was no need for a post-mortem.

Within a couple of hours of Bessie's death, Henry dispatched a telegram to Uncle Herbert, which was received at Trowbridge Post Office at 10.27 a.m. It said simply: 'Bessie died in a fit this morning letter following.' The letter, which arrived the following day, said:

Dear Sir,

Words cannot describe the great shock I suffered in the loss of my wife.

The Doctor said she had a fit in the bath and I can assure you and all her relatives that everything was done which was possible to do on her behalf. I can say no more.

Believe me,

Yours faithfully,

Henry Williams

Henry failed to inform Bessie's uncle or her brother of the date of the inquest, which took place on the 15 July, and recorded a verdict of death by misadventure, owing to a fit – in other words, accidental death. And he didn't relay the date of her funeral – the 16th – in time for them to attend. The local undertaker, Alfred Hogbin, remembered that Henry wanted an inexpensive funeral as 'it did not matter once a person had passed away, how they were buried, so long as one had done what they could for them when alive.' So Bessie's funeral was as plain and simple as her marriage had been. The modest cortège consisted of a hearse drawn by two horses, followed by a single-horse brougham, and she was buried in a common grave. The only two people to attend her funeral were Henry and the next-door-neighbour, Percy Millgate. Mr Hogbin presented his bill – £7 8s – and Henry settled within two days, but underpaid him by a shilling.

On the morning of the funeral Henry visited Carrie Rapley at the estate agent's office. He was 'trembling', she said. He 'laid his head and arms on the top of my desk and burst out sobbing', so she asked him, 'Whatever is the matter?'

He looked up at me and said 'Haven't you heard?' I said 'No what is it?' He said, 'She is dead.' I said 'Who?' He said, 'My wife.' I was very surprised, and it was quite a shock to me. I could not speak for a few moments, but a short time after I said,

'What was it?' He said 'She had been having fits, and she went
to have a bath, and she must have had another one while I was
out, and been drowned in her bath.' I said 'What bath?' He said,
'Oh it was a large one, which she bought herself, and it was put
upstairs.' He then leant his head on his arms again on the desk,
and remained in that position for a short while, when he suddenly looked up at me and said 'Wasn't it a jolly good job I got
her to make out her will.'

I was so surprised and horrified at the way he said it, at such
a sad time that I could not speak. He looked at me angrily and
said 'Well of course I did.' Then making a gesture with his hand
he said 'Isn't it the proper thing, when people are married for
the wife to make her will and leave everything to her husband,
and for the husband to make his will and leave everything to his
wife?' I then looked him straight in the eyes and said 'Did you
make yours?' He said 'Of course I did.' I said, 'But you told me
that you hadn't got anything' and he said, 'Oh well I made a
will all the same.'

Percy Millgate and his wife Ellen felt sorry for Henry. On the
day of Bessie's death they gave him dinner, and when he said he
thought he would be unable to sleep at no. 80, Ellen allowed him
to board next door. 'He could not sleep without a light,' she said
later, 'and sometimes he would go out and walk about the streets
and I would not hear him come in as he had a latch-key.' Local
policeman, Sergeant Gutteridge, saw Henry on three or four
occasions 'parading up and down the sea front in the early hours
of the morning.' He 'appeared to be very much depressed, and
on being spoken to by me, stated he could not sleep since he lost
his wife'.

A day or so after the funeral Henry visited the ironmonger
Adolphus Hill in order to negotiate the return of the bath to the
shop, and managed to persuade him to take it back for the same
price as he had paid for it – £1 17s 6d. The rest of the furniture
in the house was bought back by Alfred Hogbin, who sold

furniture when he was not busy as an undertaker. On 18 July, Henry wrote again to Uncle Herbert, telling of his shock at losing 'the one I thought more of than any one in this world.' His only comfort was 'the great God himself to whom I pray and rely for sufficient strength to bear this calamity'. After that, Uncle Herbert heard no more from Henry Williams.

2

The Young Pathologist

B ERNARD SPILSBURY WAS the same age as Bessie. Back in the summer of 1910, when they were both 33, and Bessie was taking dreamy afternoon walks and falling under the spell of Henry Williams, Spilsbury was making his name as a doctor. His life was quite different from hers. He had the authority that often comes to men blessed with good looks – he was more than six foot tall, and particularly handsome, with fine features, sensitive eyes and a strong chin.

That year, while Bessie was drifting aimlessly, Spilsbury was putting down roots. He had bought a little house in Harrow-on-the-Hill, where he lived with his wife Edith, who was pregnant with their first child. And, with Edith's support, he was working long hours, building a career. Each day he commuted into London on the Metropolitan Line and descended to the 'lower regions' of St Mary's Hospital, where he applied himself to the unfashionable specialty that he had chosen – forensic pathology. Slowly, he was gaining a reputation. He did not possess a startling intellect, or demonstrate unusual scientific flair – but his superiors had noticed that he was almost obsessively committed to his work, and was willing to devote his every waking moment to the arduous business of dissecting and analysing corpses.

The work was regarded as physically demanding, low-status and unpleasant. Knives, saws, chisels and mallets were the rougher tools of the trade, used to cut through bone and open up difficult areas such as the skull. And the equipment for putting the body back together at the end of an autopsy was similarly prosaic: needles, twine, sponges and sawdust. But Spilsbury's skills were suited to the job. He was steady and careful with a scalpel, and had a good sense of smell (though he later lost it) with which to detect the presence of poisons and other peculiarities. He undoubtedly enjoyed his work, taking on as many bodies as he could get hold of – in time, he cut up more than 25,000 of them. He wrote up many of his autopsies on hundreds of little white 'case-cards' that survive in archives in London and Nottingham.

One day he would turn his attention to Bessie's decomposing body, ruminating on the manner of her death as he subjected her torso to the criss-crossing of his blade and the probing of his forceps. But not yet. In 1910 she was still walking, and thinking and breathing fresh air, while he was shut up with death in the postmortem room. The mortuary was kept cold for hygienic reasons, and made light by the high windows and white-tiled walls. The smells of the trade were different from those of the operating theatre (blood), or the dissecting room (grease), being the sharp aroma of formaldehyde and carbolic soap, and the clinging, burning odour of the vulcanized rubber used to make mortuary aprons.

Bernard Spilsbury's intellectual energy was, year-in year-out, expended here and in the mortuaries of Paddington, Marylebone, Finchley and Hampstead, poring over the recently – and sometimes not so recently – dead, coming up with the innumerable solutions to a single question: what was the cause of death of the person laid out before him? His case-cards, covered in spindly, spidery handwritten notes, give a sense of the intensity and highly focused nature of his life, and also of the poignancy of untimely death.

A hundred years later, the incidence of death under anaesthetic seems shocking. On 11 February 1910 Spilsbury performed a post-mortem on the body of 5-year-old William Pink, who had died during an operation to straighten out the curves in his rickety legs. The following day, he recorded the same cause of death – by anaesthetic – for William Dobridge, a 15-year-old who needed an operation on his adenoids. In the following weeks and months the anaesthetic was to blame when Alice Macolino, a 7-year-old with tuberculosis, died during an abdominal operation, and 26-year-old Charlotte Parr died during surgery on her nose. Ten-week-old Herbert Wallington did not survive a routine circumcision. The killer in all these cases was chloroform – the wonder treatment that had allowed millions to undergo dental and surgical operations without pain, but which carried a fatal risk. About one in 2,500 people under anaesthetic were killed by it – ten times as many as today.

Spilsbury's 1910 case-cards also describe deaths from tetanus, like that which infected the wound on the right hand of 52-year-old George Smith, and deaths from medicines which far from curing the sick, poisoned them. The card for 46-year-old Amelia Pratt, whose body lay on his slab in January, begins with the words: 'strychnine. Accidental in medicine'. The notes on the exterior of the body record that it is 'well nourished', and rigor mortis has set in. 'Hands are clenched and livid. There are three punctures in the right forearm. The tongue is bitten on each side of the tip. There is a small abrasion on the left lower lip, and blood in the mouth.' Spilsbury's medical notes on the internal organs follow – and then a brief, staccato history of Amelia's final hours: 'Healthy but intemperate. Dec 31 Abdominal pains. Continued 2–3 days. Dr Fletcher gave bottle of medicine. Took a dose about 7.15 p.m. After a few minutes felt bad and walked about. Husband fetched home at 8.45, found her in a fit. She said medicine was burning her inside. Died 9.15 p.m.'

His cases that year included several suicides, including 46-year-old Walter Parrott, who poisoned himself with hydrochloric acid and died within 24 hours, and 18-year-old George Snow, who swallowed hydrocyanic acid. The cause of death of

Beatrice O'Connor, aged 45, is put down to 'Coal gas poisoning. Suicide'. Spilsbury writes that she was 'brought in by police who found her in locked room and gas stove turned on'.

There was a steady stream of deaths of women from criminal abortions. Florence Warren, who was 22, became pregnant by a man 'to whom she had been engaged for two years'. She visited an illegal abortionist, Mrs Cullen, 'to get her out of her trouble', and died after a miscarriage and several days in great pain. Elsie Hertzog died that summer, aged 21, after a back-street abortion, and a 40-year-old spinster, Kate Balderson, a district nurse, died of a haemorrhage after attempting a home abortion with a knitting needle.

Then there were the autopsies on infants. Spilsbury records that seven-week-old Cicely Kisk died from starvation. 'Mother said child became suddenly unconscious on day of admission', he wrote. 'Quite well prior to this. History doubted owing to extreme emaciation of child.' Two months earlier the body of another baby lay before him:

> child unknown. Female . . . Mummified. Face sunken. Eyes gone . . . Heart thin and papery. Lungs papery . . . Liver, Kidneys, Bladder, Stomach and intestines distinguishable but thin and parchment like. Other organs not distinguished . . . found in lost luggage dept London Bridge Ry Station on Feb 16 1910. Sent from Victoria Stn on Dec 9 1909. Parcel left at Victoria Stn 10 Nov 1908. Child lay on left side in cardboard box. Face was downwards and partly covered by piece of black cloth.

He arrives at no conclusion for the death of this nameless child, writing only: 'stillborn?'

It was hard toil, but there was, increasingly, a public reward for the doctors who were prepared to dedicate their lives to this grisly business. Every so often a big murder trial came their way, and the flashes of the press cameras and the spectacle of the courtroom instantly compensated for the everyday litany of death and the confines of the mortuary. When the forensic pathologist left the hospital for the public stage, and took the role of 'expert witness', he was transformed into a powerful figure who might, through his evidence, set a man free or send him to the gallows. As Bernard Spilsbury knew, though, there was an inherent difficulty that came with the role – and that was the newness, and so the fragility, of the expert medical witness as figure of authority. For the past fifty years the British had distrusted the forensic pathologist in the courtroom.

The underlying problem went back to mid-Victorian times, and the 1859 trial of Dr Thomas Smethurst for the murder of Isabella Bankes. Dr Smethurst had married Isabella bigamously, and tended her when shortly afterwards she became pregnant and was desperately ill with vomiting and diarrhoea. The efforts of her physician, Dr Julius, brought about no improvement. In fact she got considerably worse – and when her life seemed to be slipping away Dr Julius suspected that Isabella had been poisoned. On 1 May 1859 he sent a stool sample for investigation. Arsenic was found, and an antidote administered. But Isabella did not respond, and died on 3 May. Dr Smethurst was arrested the same day.

The trial became a national sensation, and produced an unedifying display of medical men at war. Ten doctors testified that she was poisoned, and seven that she died from natural causes. The vital testimony in the case came from Britain's most highly regarded forensic pathologist, who was among the ten doctors who appeared as witnesses for the prosecution. Dr Alfred Swaine Taylor was a lecturer in medical jurisprudence at Guy's Hospital, London, and the author of world-renowned standard textbooks on medical jurisprudence and poisons. In his early fifties, he was at the peak of his career, and an established figure in prominent murder trials. It was he who had tested the stool sample and found arsenic. In court, however, he admitted that he had made a mistake during the test. The arsenic had come *not* from the sample, but from the copper gauze that he had used during his experiment. His professional rivals, unsurprisingly, were quick to testify that that there was no evidence at all for arsenic poisoning. But, to the astonishment of many – including the press – Dr Taylor did not change his conclusion. The test may have been faulty, he said, but he still believed that Isabella Bankes had died from arsenic poisoning.

The judge, in his summing-up, seemed to accept Dr Taylor's opinion. He was a close friend of Taylor, which may or may not have influenced his view. But, perhaps more significant, was the extraordinary status of the doctor. Expert witnesses for the Crown generally enjoyed a respect that defence witnesses did not. And of the Crown witnesses, Alfred Swaine Taylor was the most senior of all – renowned for his particular expertise in poisons. In any case, the jury was sufficiently impressed to find Dr Smethurst guilty, and he was sentenced to hang.

A huge outcry in the medical press and national newspapers followed. An editorial in the *British Medical Journal* deplored Dr Taylor's 'lamentable error':

> If . . . the man who holds in his hands the keys of life and death will not insist upon purity in his tests, then we say that the horrors which flourished in the days of witchcraft, when human life hung upon the lips of any old crone, will be but too faithfully represented by the horrors which will flow from the pseudo-scientific evidence of the present day.

Under pressure, the Home Secretary, Sir Lewis Cornewall, took advice from an eminent surgeon, Sir Benjamin Brodie, on whether the conviction was safe. Soon afterwards, a letter from the Home Secretary appeared in *The Times*, stating that Dr Smethurst was to receive a pardon. The wrong verdict, he thought, had come about not because of any fault in British criminal tribunals but because of 'the imperfection of medical science, and from the fallibility of judgement' of doctors. Dr Taylor's career was now in decline, and the reputation of forensic pathology was in shreds.

Twenty years later, a trial in America proved similarly disastrous for the reputation of forensic scientists there. The body of a young woman named Mary Stannard was found in Rockland, Connecticut, with bruises on her head and her throat cut. After the burial, rumours spread that a local Methodist minister, Herbert Hayden, had made Mary pregnant and subsequently killed her. He was arrested, and Mary's half-sister told the authorities that Herbert Hayden possessed a knife that was stained with blood. This opened up a debate that had been raging for half a century – would the scientists be able to determine whether the blood on Hayden's knife belonged to a human or an animal? Experts were brought in and promptly disagreed about the evidence. The prosecution now changed its approach. Hayden had admitted buying arsenic in order to poison rats; so Mary's body was exhumed, and the state forensic pathologist Professor Moses White, of Yale College, found fifty grains of arsenic in the stomach – enough to kill not just one person, but many.

Amongst the 176 witnesses in the trial that opened in October 1879 were 'twelve distinguished professors, eight of them from Yale college, and fifteen doctors of all grades and shapes'. They lined up against each other on three core questions – whether an ovarian tumour found during the autopsy would have caused Mary to think she was pregnant, the significance of the arsenic, and the nature of the blood on the knife. The scene was one of utter confusion as the experts disagreed about everything and the jury failed to reach a verdict. The Revd Hayden was again a free man, and science once more discredited. The *New York Times* put it succinctly:

It is not necessary to impute dishonesty or mercenary motives to
the eminent experts in medicine or other branches of science

whose disagreements put the minds of jurymen in a maze, instead of leading them into the light. But there are experts and experts, there are theories and theories, and there are even facts and facts, in every department of science or special knowledge, and lawyers can ingeniously make their selection, giving prominence to some and keeping others out of sight, and twisting and turning until the inexpert mind in the jury box is in danger of losing all faith in science as a witness.

By 1910 memories of Alfred Swaine Taylor had subsided. People had forgotten the danger that arose when expert witnesses gained too much power in the courtroom, when an individual's influence went beyond his scientific competence. And at St Mary's hospital the forensic team was busy rebuilding the credibility of 'science as a witness'. That July they received a telephone call from the Home Office asking for a doctor to attend a house at 39 Hilldrop Crescent, Camden, where some body parts had been found in the cellar. The most senior pathologist at the hospital, Augustus Pepper, went to the scene, accompanied by Chief Inspector Walter Dew of Scotland Yard. Bernard Spilsbury was still in the second rank and so stayed behind.

When he arrived, Dr Pepper was greeted by an overpowering stench. The police had removed bricks from the floor of the cellar exposing a mass of soapy gloop, barely recognizable as human. The doctor crouched down and conducted an examination at the site, identifying 'a large piece of flesh, composed of skin, fat and muscle, that came from the thigh and lower part of the buttock', and a number of organs – 'the viscera of the chest and abdomen in one piece, that is the heart, the lungs, the lower two and a half inches of the windpipe, the gullet, the liver, the kidneys, spleen, stomach, pancreas'.

The body had been filleted in such a way as to make identification almost impossible. The head was missing, and so were the limbs and genitalia. Pepper inspected the soil, and found that it had lime mixed into it. In addition, 'I found some articles in the hole, some of these were taken from the hole and put on a tray. Among them there was a tuft of brown hair in a Hinde's curler . . . The natural colour of the hair was dark brown; the part in the curler showed graduations of bleaching.' He also found a handkerchief and some pieces of clothing.

The following day, 15 July 1910, Augustus Pepper made a further examination of the body parts, which had now been removed from the cellar and taken to Islington mortuary. He found twenty pubic hairs, some of which were still attached to the skin, and also recorded 'another piece of skin, 7 inches by 6 inches, which came from the lower part, the front portion of the abdomen'. There was, he said later, 'a mark upon that piece that attracted my attention, and I afterwards examined it with particularity. I spent several hours examining it.' The mark was possibly a scar, of about four inches in length. The findings in the cellar were put into five jars, and kept for further examination. Dr Pepper had it in mind to ask his colleagues William Willcox and the promising junior, Bernard Spilsbury, for their opinions.

In the meantime, the story of the body parts was becoming a national and international news story. No. 39 Hilldrop Crescent was the home of Hawley Harvey Crippen, an American living in England and earning a living as a homeopathic doctor who also sold 'patent medicines' – the branded pills and remedies despised by the medical profession but advertised everywhere, and supposed to cure practically anything.

It was a large, sombre house, in a road not far from Holloway prison. Crippen had lived there with his wife, Cora, a big, blousy woman who, using the name Belle Elmore, had tried and failed to make a career as a music-hall singer. They made an odd couple; she was loud and bossy, while he seemed unassuming and submissive. While she dolled up her voluptuous body in jewels, furs and fancy clothes, he was an unprepossessing sight – ugly, balding, weak-chinned and goggle-eyed. 'In looking at him,' said his friend Seymour Hicks, 'I was by no means sure I was not talking to a bream or a mullet.' In public, and private, Cora treated her husband with contempt.

In February 1910 Cora suddenly went missing, and Crippen moved his mistress of three years, Ethel le Neve, into the house. Crippen told Cora's friends that she had gone back to America, and in March he said she had died there of pneumonia. But the friends were not convinced, and when Ethel started going about wearing Cora's jewellery, the police were called in. On 9 July Crippen and Ethel fled London, and police notices quickly went up all over the country: 'Wanted for murder and mutilation of a woman; Hawley Harvey Crippen . . . long sandy moustache, rather straggly, may be clean shaven or wearing beard; eyes grey; flat on bridge of nose; false teeth . . . throws his feet out when walking; speaks with slight American accent; wears hat on back of head . . .' A description of Ethel was also issued: 'Complexion pale, hair light brown; large grey eyes; good teeth; good looking; pleasant appearance; quiet subdued manner; looks intently when in conversation; walks slowly; reticent; probably dressed blue serge suit, grey hard felt hat; or may be dressed as a boy in dark brown suit.' The instruction went out to police to watch railway stations and docks, and to search outgoing ships. According to the front page of the *Daily Express*, 60,000 policemen had joined the hunt.

It soon emerged that the couple had escaped the country by a cross-channel ferry, and taken refuge at the Hôtel des Ardennes in Brussels. The *Daily Mirror* sent a reporter to the spot, but by the time he arrived, Crippen and Ethel had moved on, once again boarding a ship. The paper devoted its front page to a picture of the glum-looking proprietress of the Ardennes, 'Madame Vital', alongside a photograph of 'Crippen's favourite seat at the hotel'.

Crippen and Ethel were unaware of the incredible manhunt, and did not realize that they were just one step ahead of the press and the police. According to Ethel, they were in good spirits as they boarded the SS *Montrose*, bound for Quebec, registering as Mr John Robinson and Master Robinson – father and son. Unluckily for them, the ship's captain, a dashing young man named Henry Kendall, had, on the day of the ship's departure, bought a copy of the continental edition of the *Daily Mail*, and was up to date on all the details of the 'North London Cellar Murder'. Three hours after they set off, he took a stroll about the deck of the *Montrose*, and noticed 'Mr and Master Robinson' walking together, holding hands in a way that suggested a particular intimacy. When Master Robinson gave his father's hand a squeeze, Captain Kendall thought the gesture 'strange and unnatural'. He paused to take a closer look at the couple, wished them a pleasant morning, and moved on. Without further hesitation, he ordered the ship's stewards to lock away all the newspapers on board and went to his cabin, where he retrieved his revolver, and put it in his pocket.

Henry Kendall allowed more than a day to pass without contacting the police. He wanted to be sure that his suspicions were correct, and confided in his first officer, Alfred Sargent, who then inspected the Robinsons. The fact was that Ethel, despite having allowed Crippen to cut her hair, did not make a convincing boy. It did not help matters that the seat of her trousers had split under pressure, and was held together with safety-pins. Sargent thought them odd, and agreed that they could be Hawley Crippen and Ethel le Neve. Captain Kendall realized that if he were going to alert the police, he had to do it soon. The Marconi wireless telegraph on board the *Montrose* had a range of 150 miles, and would be useless once they were in the middle of the Atlantic.

In the afternoon of Friday 22 July he sent for Llewellyn Jones, who was employed by the Marconi company and acted as the ship's wireless operator. Jones relayed a message in Morse code:

Have strong suspicions that Crippen London Cellar Murderer and accomplice are amongst saloon passengers. Moustache taken off growing beard. Accomplice dressed as boy voice manner and build undoubtedly a girl. Both travelling as Mr and Master Robinson. Kendall.

The communication was instantly portrayed as a wonder of modern science. The deployment of wireless telegraphy in tracking down a murderer made the front page of newspapers on both sides of the Atlantic, and all around the world. In France, the *Liberté* expressed the common view that the new technology 'has demonstrated that from one side of the Atlantic to the other a criminal lives in a cage of glass, where he is much more exposed to the eyes of the public than if he remained on land'. The papers now avidly reported the latest news each day, as Chief Inspector Walter Dew boarded another ship, the SS *Laurentic*, with a view to overtaking the *Montrose* and arresting Crippen and Ethel le Neve before they set foot in Canada.

The newspapers published charts of the Atlantic Ocean, tracking the estimated positions of the two ships. On board the *Montrose*, Captain Kendall was inundated by more than fifty marconigrams from newspapers in Britain, America and Canada, enquiring after Crippen and Ethel. Was the doctor disguised as a clergyman? Had the couple been arrested yet? The *New York World* was the most audacious, sending a wire addressed to Crippen with the message: 'Will gladly print all you will say.'

At midnight on 27 July, the *Laurentic* overtook the *Montrose*, and Chief Inspector Dew arrived in Canada ahead of his quarry, to be greeted by the clamour of the news-hungry press. Dew refused all requests for interviews, and instead insisted on being rowed out to meet the *Montrose*, where he arrested Crippen and Ethel. Within days, he was escorting them back across the Atlantic, and when they arrived in Liverpool on Saturday, 27 August, it was to the boos and jeers of a crowd of many hundreds who were waiting at the docks. Crippen suddenly confessed that he could not face the ordeal ahead, and Dew lent him his own heavy Ulster overcoat, which covered him from head to toe. 'When all was ready we made a dash for the waiting train', wrote Dew, 'facing a battery of cameras as we made our way down the gangway.' But as they drew into Euston, it became clear that the crowds there were even more antagonistic than those at Liverpool. The boos could be heard before the train had drawn to a stand-still.

The little party was now driven to Bow Street Police Station. Dew reported:

> another tremendous crowd . . . More boos and more jeers. The police had taken every precaution. This was just as well, for an ugly rush was made towards the cab in which Crippen and I were travelling. Fortunately, the double gates leading to the rear of the station had been opened and we dashed through. The gates were then slammed in the faces of the angry mob.

On the morning of 29 August, Hawley Crippen and Ethel le Neve appeared, side by side, in the dock at Bow Street police court. Somewhere inside the courtroom a reporter took a secret photograph, some say from a camera hidden inside his hat. It shows Crippen solemn, but alert, looking like a sad weasel – his infamous bulging eyes drooping mournfully, his face heavy with melancholy. Ethel, on his left side, was swamped by her thick serge suit and large hat secured with a veil. Her eyes were cast down and her face gaunt. The picture suggests a new phase in the Crippen story. Now that he had been captured, the world wanted to know the details of what had happened to Cora. How did he kill her? And, given that there were no witnesses (the police were increasingly convinced that Ethel was, at most, an accessory after the fact), how was murder to be proven? In short, would the forensic scientists be able to piece together the truth – not just a hazy, balance-of-probabilities sort of truth, but an unequivocal rendition of the facts which would stand up in court?

The first and most obvious challenge for the Crown was to amass evidence that the remains found in the cellar were, indeed, parts of the body of Cora Crippen. Without the head and genitalia, this was not going to be easy. (One theory was that Crippen had put Cora's head in a bag and, during his Easter holiday, had dropped it overboard from a cross-channel ferry.) The hair found in the Hinde curler was up to eight inches long, too long for a man, and was dark at the roots, but otherwise bleached. This was consistent with the way in which Cora treated her hair. But it was not conclusive – many women bleached their hair. The undergarments found at the scene were women's, and of the type that Cora favoured. But this evidence was less relevant than a rotting pyjama-jacket that was also found in the soil beneath the cellar.

A breakthrough came when Walter Dew attended the formal inquest into the death of Cora Crippen.

> After the proceedings were over I was standing idly outside the court close to a group of women who were discussing the case. One of the women was Mrs Paul Martinetti, who had been a close friend of Belle Elmore (Cora), and I pricked up my ears when I overheard her say something about Belle having undergone a serious operation. I called Mrs Martinetti to one side and asked her if I had heard all right. 'Oh yes,' she replied. 'Belle had an operation years ago in America. She had quite a big scar on the lower part of her body. I have seen it.' Here was something really vital. If that scar could be found on those gruesome remnants of human flesh lying in the Islington mortuary it might provide the missing link in the chain of evidence of identification.

He relayed the information to 'one of the medical men in the case', and on 8 August, at St Mary's, Dr Pepper invited his colleague William Willcox to examine the tissue. Willcox supported Pepper's view that the hairs at one end of the skin were pubic hair. He made notes on his observations, and 'put the skin in a special fluid designed to prevent further changes of putrefaction'. Pepper now suggested that Spilsbury should take a look at the specimen. Two years earlier Pepper had proposed that the younger man make a detailed study of scars and scar tissue, and his resulting expertise could now be critical.

Bernard Spilsbury first saw the piece of skin on 9 September and formed the opinion that it came from the lower part of the wall of the abdomen, near the middle. 'I base that opinion on the presence and arrangement of certain muscles,' he later told the jury at the Old Bailey, 'besides that there is a row of short, dark hairs at the lower margin of the piece, those hairs being in my opinion pubic hairs.' He next examined sections from the skin under the microscope, and while he found glands in some parts of the segment, he 'found no glands in the centre where there is the mark called a scar, proving in fact that mark is a scar . . . As the result of my microscopical examination,' he concluded, 'I say that mark is undoubtedly an old operation scar.'

Thus, Spilsbury's view was entirely consistent with the remains in the cellar at 39 Hilldrop Crescent being those of Cora Crippen, whose operation scar had been exactly at that point – on her lower abdomen. No one seemed bothered that Spilsbury and his colleagues had been informed of Cora's operation scar *before* they examined the piece of skin with the strange mark.

That summer, the police also established that some time around 17 or 18 January 1910, shortly before Cora had gone missing, Dr Crippen had bought five grains of a substance called hyoscine hydrobromide from the Lewis and Burrows chemist on New Oxford Street in London. Charles Hetherington, who served him, said later that he had never known the chemist to keep such a large quantity of hyoscine in stock, and he had had to order it in from the supplier. Crippen had been a regular customer of the shop, but this was the first time that he had asked for hyoscine, a drug derived from the nightshade group of plants, which is poisonous in anything other than tiny doses.

Hyoscine, these days, is used in minute quantities to treat travel sickness and post-operative nausea, and to dilate the pupil of the eye. In 1910, according to William Willcox, it was used as a powerful sedative – the proper dose being between one-hundredth to one two-hundredth of a grain, so Crippen had bought enough for at least five hundred doses. In fact, he told Charles Hetherington that he had bought it for 'homeopathic purposes'. If that were true, he had ordered enough to treat the population of a small town. Dr Crippen's story didn't seem credible – and neither the English nor American pharmacopoeias of the time contain any reference to hyoscine as a homeopathic remedy.

On 2 August William Willcox, at St Mary's, was told that Crippen had purchased hyoscine. He then began a series of tests on the stomach, intestines, kidney and liver, which were contained in the five glass storage jars. 'I tested for all the common alkaloids,' he said, 'morphia, strychnine, cocaine and so on,' and found that a mydriatic alkaloid was present – mydriatic meaning that the substance will dilate a pupil. This he tested by squirting it into the eye of a cat. Further tests narrowed the options, until Willcox was left with one result – he had found the presence of hyoscine in the body parts. He said that he had found in the organs two-fifths of a grain, which 'would certainly correspond to more than half a grain in the whole body' – an amount which would, he said, be a fatal dose. Again, nobody seemed disturbed by the fact that Willcox had known of Crippen's purchase of hyoscine *before* commencing his experiments.

Willcox later described the effects of the poison: 'It would perhaps produce a little delirium and excitement at first; the pupils of the eyes would be paralysed; the mouth and the throat would be dry, and then quickly the patient would become drowsy and unconscious and completely paralysed, and death would result in a few hours.' This, he said, was the first time that he had ever found hyoscine in a dead body, and the first time that he had ever known hyoscine to be connected to a case of murder.

The biggest breakthrough in the case came late in the day. For some reason, that summer Chief Inspector Dew failed to investigate the significance of the portion of pyjama-jacket that was found with the human remains at Hilldrop Crescent. The jacket, which had been wrapped around some of the body parts, bore the label 'Jones Brothers' – a well-known draper's and outfitter's with a shop on the Holloway Road. The prosecution lawyers in the case, Richard Muir and Travers Humphreys, both exasperated by Dew's inaction, decided to turn detective themselves, and sent a list of questions to be put to 'a responsible representative of the company'.

The reply was revelatory – the lawyers were assured by the company's buyer that the jacket was part of an order from 39 Hilldrop Crescent, in January 1909, for three sets of pyjamas. The remaining two sets and the missing trousers from the third set were all found in the Crippens' house. This, the lawyers agreed, proved beyond doubt that the human remains were placed in the cellar while Crippen was living in the house, not before. By the time that Dr Crippen came to trial, on 18 October 1910, the prosecution lawyers were confident that they had amassed enough evidence to convict him. Crowds filled the streets outside the Old Bailey, and men and women in their millions purchased the newspapers that were full of the sort of story they liked best – a good, old-fashioned murder.

Across London, a drama of a not so different sort was being staged. In August 1910 a Sherlock Holmes story, *The Speckled Band*, had opened at the Adelphi Theatre, transferred to the Globe in September, and was still attracting strong audiences. (In October it would open in Boston, and in November in New York.) The story features a cold-hearted man, Dr Rylott, who, motivated by financial gain, appears to have murdered his step-daughter, Julia. There being no witnesses to his evil deed, it falls to Sherlock Holmes to work out, through his powers of observation and deduction, how Julia died. The great detective is, as usual, successful, and establishes that Rylott has released a venomous snake into Julia's room at night. He proves his contention by allowing Rylott to attempt another murder – this time of Julia's sister Helen – intervening just in time to attack the snake, and send it out of the room. When the angry snake bites and kills Rylott it is clear that the powers of one man's rigorous, scientific approach to crime have brought about justice – albeit of the rougher sort.

Sherlock Holmes was the embodiment of the medical detective: the man of science who could outwit the criminal. As yet there was no real-life Sherlock Holmes, but the fictional medical detective was massively popular. The public adored the idea that crimes might be solved by the ingenious application of a logical mind. Not just any mind, but one that had been almost entirely stripped of sentiment and weakness in order to become a magnificent scientific instrument, an alliance of intelligence, deductive powers, perception and medical knowledge. There remained just enough sentiment to allow Holmes to make occasional mistakes or suddenly to display emotion. Apart from a love of cocaine and playing the violin, he had few other human interests. He did not fall in love all the time, have a failed marriage or psychological issues to wrestle with. The creator of Holmes, Sir Arthur Conan Doyle, regularly acknowledged that the chief inspiration for his detective came from the medical world, in the form of the Edinburgh surgeon Joseph Bell.

Conan Doyle, who was a doctor himself, had attended Bell's lectures and been struck by his teacher's extraordinary instant diagnoses of patients, based on keen observation. Bell claimed to be able to tell that one patient was an army man, serving in a Highland Regiment in the West Indies, simply from his bearing, his accent and the nature of his complaint. He astonished another of his patients by observing 'You came from Liberton . . . You drive two horses, one grey and one bay, you are probably employed by a brewery.' Later Bell told his students: 'I saw the clay from Liberton on the fellow's boots. He had grey hairs on one sleeve and bay hairs on the other. As for my final bit of deduction, you probably observed the face, especially the nose.'

In 1901 Conan Doyle wrote:

It was my own good fortune to have found the qualities of my hero in actual life . . . I saw and heard the ease with which my teacher reasoned from points which were hardly visible to me, and arrived at just conclusions from the most trivial details. There grew upon me the conviction that the resources of the human brain in this direction had never been appreciated, and that a scientific system might give results more remarkable than any of the arbitrary and inexplicable triumphs which so often fall to the lot of the detective in fiction.

Two weeks before the Crippen trial opened, Conan Doyle gave an address at St Mary's Hospital. It was wonderful to note, he said, the progress in medicine during the past thirty years. 'This generation had,' he thought, 'brought about a greater change in medical science than any century had done before. At last there was some attempt to make it exact . . .' He took the opportunity of observing the 'exactness' of the medical evidence against Crippen by attending the trial.

The prosecution was led by Richard Muir, a formidable Scotsman who was known for his meticulous preparation and his grasp of detail. On hearing that Muir had taken the case, Crippen said: 'I wish it had been anyone else. I fear the worst.' Muir had worked out that the trial would become a battle between the expert witnesses for the defence, and the expert witnesses for the prosecution – that is, one set of scientists against another. He was relying on the strength of evidence supplied by the doctors at St Mary's.

The team was led by Augustus Pepper, who described the remains that had been found in Dr Crippen's cellar. Judging by the way in which the internal organs – or viscera – had been removed, he said, 'I think it must have been done by a person skilled in removing viscera – skilled in dissection.' On the critical question of the scar, he admitted under cross-examination that when he had first examined the body parts, he did not see the relevant mark on the flesh, and that later, when he did find the scar, he had already learned of Cora Crippen's operation. He also acknowledged that medical science did not allow him to state how long the body parts had been in the cellar, and admitted that much of the flesh had been 'converted into a kind of soap' due to the presence of damp clay in the soil under 39 Hilldrop Crescent.

Bernard Spilsbury was the next of the St Mary's doctors to appear for the prosecution. He stood out instantly being younger than his colleagues and altogether more striking in appearance – taller, more attractive and impeccably turned out. When he spoke, he was clearer and more succinct. 'I have on several occasions examined the piece of skin and flesh,' he said, 'the first time on September 9. It comes from the lower part of the wall of the abdomen, near the middle line. I base that opinion upon the presence and the arrangement of certain muscles.' He also made particular mention of a tendon attached to those muscles.

> On 9 September I made a section across the middle of what I regard as a scar and examined it under the microscope. There was no epidermis on the surface of the mark, but I found a small mass embedded deeply in it at one spot. This indicates to me the line of incision of the skin at the operation which caused the scar. At each end of the section on either side of the scar there were glands, but there were no glands on the scar itself . . . The mark is undoubtedly an old operation scar.

Under cross-examination, Spilsbury supported Augustus Pepper, stating that that the person who had removed the viscera 'must have had considerable dexterity and considerable anatomical knowledge'. He also admitted that he had known that Cora Crippen had had an operation when he first examined the skin. Re-examined by the prosecution he said, loud and clear: 'It is beyond doubt that this is a scar . . . There is in my opinion, no room for doubt that the mark was a scar.'

Spilsbury's colleague William Willcox then told the court of the experiments that he had conducted, which resulted in the identification of hyoscine in several organs of the body. Under cross-examination, he admitted that he had been aware that Crippen had purchased hyoscine before he commenced his investigation. Arthur Luff was the last of the St Mary's team to appear. He supported Willcox who, he said, had conducted 'exactly the right tests . . . The poison present was undoubtedly hyoscine, judging by those tests.'

This was the end of the forensic evidence for the prosecution. But before the defence's expert witnesses appeared, Hawley Harvey Crippen took the stand. Until then, he had been sitting quite still, listening attentively to the evidence but showing no emotion. If anything, he seemed like a well-behaved schoolboy in class, and rather likeable. It was one of the features of his trial that almost all the witnesses who knew him personally had good things to say about him, even those appearing for the prosecution. He was repeatedly described as 'a kind and amiable man'. Cora Crippen's friend Adeline Harrison thought him 'a good husband'. Ethel le Neve's landlady, Emily Jackson, said 'he was one of the nicest men I had ever met', and his business colleague Gilbert Rylance observed that even after Cora's disappearance at the beginning of February 'he showed no trace of uneasiness . . . there was no trace of abruptness; he was as kind as ever.'

Now the little doctor spoke for the first time. At first, he said, he had been 'on friendly terms' with his wife, 'but she was always rather hasty in her temper' and, after a while, 'she was always finding fault with me, and every night took the opportunity of quarrelling with me, so that we went to bed in rather a temper with each other.' She had, he said, taken up with another man – by the name of Bruce Miller. After that, 'I still lived with her – not as my wife, but I still lived with her.' At Hilldrop Crescent they slept in different rooms. 'Before friends and strangers', said Crippen, 'it was always agreed that we should treat each other as if there had never been any trouble'. However, Cora got into rages and tempers. These were generally 'over very trivial matters; she was always finding fault with trivial things.'

There was, in fact, some public sympathy for someone who appeared to be a mild-mannered, kind-hearted man, trapped in a hellish marriage with a hypercritical harridan of a woman. The journalist Filson Young expressed the common view neatly: 'Crippen was not a robust man physically', he wrote, 'his vitality was of a nervous sort. She, on the other hand, was robust and animal. Her vitality was of that loud, aggressive, and physical kind that seems to exhaust the atmosphere round it, and is exhausting to live with.' Many people were inclined to think that if justice were done, Crippen would not hang.

Much now depended on the performance of the expert witnesses for the defence. These gentlemen were doctors from the London Hospital, and rivals of the St Mary's team. First to take the witness stand was Gilbert Turnbull, who was director of the hospital's Pathological Institute. Under his supervision, he said, the London team conducted more than 1,200 post-mortems a year. He also spent his time examining under the microscope material that was sent to him each day by the hospital's surgeons. He had seen the piece of flesh said to contain a scar on three occasions. 'My microscopical examination of the specimens enables me to say,' he told the court, 'that what has been called a scar cannot possibly be one. The grounds of my opinion are that I find certain structures which have never been found in a scar before.' He had identified, he said, some hair follicles and traces of a sebaceous gland – which would not be present in scar tissue. He thought the mark in the skin had been made not by a surgeon's scalpel but by 'the skin having been folded over and something having been between the fold, and thus producing pressure, which dried the skin at the fold.'

Under cross-examination, though, Gilbert Turnbull's appearance of certainty began to crumble. He admitted that he had first formed the opinion that the flesh was not from the abdomen, but after having read the reports of Spilsbury and his colleagues, was no longer sure. He stated that he had not seen the tendon mentioned by Spilsbury. The court witnessed the body parts being shown to Dr Turnbull, while the young, elegant Bernard Spilsbury stepped forward to point out the crucial tendon. The witness now prevaricated, and eventually said, yes, this was the tendon. The embarrassment of the London Hospital doctor was deepened further by his acknowledgement that he had only given his opinion to the defence on the strict understanding that he would not be called as a witness – a deal that had been broken by the defence solicitor, Arthur Newton. Where the alleged scar was concerned, Dr Turnbull now seemed unsure of whether he could or could not detect the presence of sebaceous glands. When he eventually repeated that 'from start to finish I have never wavered in my opinion that the mark is not a scar,' his authority was gone.

His London Hospital colleague Reginald Glyne Wall next agreed that the mark was not a scar, while a toxicologist, Alexander Blyth, disagreed with William Willcox's analysis of hyoscine found in the body parts. The jury now said that they themselves would like to inspect the flesh closely. In an adjoining room, Augustus Pepper of St Mary's pointed out what he believed to be a scar, and also a white line running down its centre which, he said was the mark of the surgeon's knife. Dr Turnbull told the jury that the white line was simply the apex of a fold in the skin. Asked to explain how the portion of the skin could have been rolled over twice, Dr Turnbull said it 'might have been done in the throwing of earth over the remains,' while Augustus Pepper stuck to his opinion that it was 'quite impossible' that the skin could have been folded twice.

In his closing speech the prosecution counsel, Richard Muir, made much of the pyjama-jacket that had been found wrapped around the body parts. This, it had been shown, belonged to Crippen. That aside, all his emphasis lay on the forensic evidence, and the mistakes that the London Hospital doctors, in particular Turnbull, had made in the witness-box, which, he said, amounted to 'confessions of incapacity or the grossest carelessness and rashness.' In his summing up the judge made it abundantly clear that it was the duty of the gentlemen of the jury to be sure, on the evidence, that the body in the cellar was that of Cora Crippen. If they were not sure, her husband was entitled to walk from the court a free man.

At 2.15 on the afternoon of Saturday, 22 October 1910, the jury retired, returning to the court in less than half an hour. The foreman said the jury was unanimous in finding the prisoner guilty of wilful murder. When asked if he would like to say anything, Crippen answered: 'I still protest my innocence.' He was hanged at Pentonville prison on 23 November 1910.

Crippen had aroused a strange mix of emotions. The public were fascinated by a man who appeared to be good and kind, and who displayed a touching loyalty to the love of his life, Ethel le Neve (who was tried separately and found not guilty). And yet the jury had been convinced that not only had he poisoned his wife, but he had carefully cut up, dissected and buried her body. On the one hand he was a monster, on the other he seemed so familiar and ordinary. The despair he must have felt at being trapped in an unhappy marriage was so easy to relate to. Divorce in 1910 was such a disgraceful act, that it regularly made front-page news – and murder could, in fiction at least, be an acceptable alternative. In the same year that he attended the Crippen trial, Sir Arthur Conan Doyle, published a story – *The Devil's Foot* – in which Sherlock Holmes allowed a murderer to walk free because he felt sympathy for a man, trapped in a bad marriage, who killed out of love for another woman. And in 1904 he had published *The Adventure of the Abbey Grange*, in which the lover of Mary Brackenstall kills her abusive husband. Again, Holmes decides, out of sympathy, to let the murderer off the hook.

Conan Doyle's friend, the barrister Edward Marshall Hall, watched the Crippen trial from the wings and was similarly sensitive to the pain of an unhappy marriage. His first wife, Ethel, had told him on their wedding day that she did not care for him and never could. He was deeply in love with her, and on his honeymoon in Paris wrote in his diary, 'I wish I were dead. Words can never tell my grief.' The marriage lasted only a few short years, before Ethel left. She died shortly afterwards, in terrible circumstances, after a botched backstreet abortion. Now, a quarter of a century later, Marshall Hall took the view that had he represented Hawley Crippen, he would have persuaded the jury that Crippen was innocent – that Cora had died not because of her husband's murderous intent, but because, under pressure from her unreasonable demands, he made a fatal error.

He would have taken the line, he said, that Crippen had not, as he claimed, ceased to have a sexual relationship with Cora. Instead he was struggling to satisfy her abnormally voracious sexual appetite. And, 'devoted as he was to his mistress', he 'found himself the victim of a double demand to which the poor little man's frail physique and advancing years rendered him unequal'. So he hit on the idea of giving her a few doses of hyoscine, knowing that it was 'sometimes used as a sexual depressant in cases of acute nymphomania'. By mistake, he got the dose wrong and when she died, he panicked, hid her body and ran away with Ethel.

There are many faults in Marshall Hall's theory, not least that Crippen himself insisted, perhaps for Ethel's benefit, that he and Cora no longer had a sexual relationship. Nonetheless, it is interesting because it presents a picture of a different sort of trial altogether – one in which the science presented by the doctors at St Mary's would come up against the artistry of a first-class lawyer who could command a courtroom, who could sway a jury with emotion and theatricality. The writer Edward Marjoribanks listened to his friend Marshall Hall setting out his plan of action· for the Crippen case. At the end, wrote Marjoribanks, 'I began to be carried away and to see Dr Crippen . . . not as a sordid and cold-blooded murderer, but as a martyr and a hero of romance . . . and I could not help thinking that, whatever William Willcox and Bernard Spilsbury might have said about hyoscine, twelve reasonable men might have preferred to believe Edward Marshall Hall.' In other words, that twelve reasonable men might be persuaded by a talented advocate that the science on offer was not to be trusted.

3

Alice

ALICE BURNHAM WAS a happy young woman of 25. She had a pretty face, and was blessed with a soft, English-rose complexion, a mass of thick hair and large smiling eyes. True, she was short – just five foot and half an inch – and she was undoubtedly overweight. But these physical deficiencies did not make her unattractive since they were easily offset by her good features and a sunny, optimistic personality. Her sister Elizabeth described her as 'always healthy and bright'.

Alice had enjoyed a solid, stable childhood, growing up in the Buckinghamshire village of Aston Clinton, where the Burnhams were one of the leading families. Thirty-three Burnhams were living in the village at the time of the 1911 census. The men were farmers or, like Alice's father Charles, coal merchants, while most of the women were housewives. And the names of three Burnham boys are to be found on the village memorial to the dead of the First World War. Alfred and Ronald were slightly younger than Alice. Andrew Burnham, who was killed in action at the Somme, was the same age.

The family were great supporters of the local Baptist church, and so Alice grew up in a close-knit Christian household. Her sister Annie said she and Alice were 'always on the best of terms and the greatest of friends'. She attended the village school, which was financed by the Rothschild family, and when the time came for her to leave, she decided to take up teaching, helping out with the local infants. It might have been necessary for her to work, since her family was not well off, but her subsequent actions suggest that money was not the only consideration. She wanted to make something of her life.

Sometime around 1906, Alice went to Aylesbury to study at the pupil-teachers' centre for a qualification that would allow her to teach older children and to earn more money. She passed two examinations but failed a third, so instead of realizing her ambitions she went back to looking after small children, taking a job as a nursery governess. However, her setback in teaching appears to have focused her mind on a change of direction, and she soon left her position and went to Hitchin General Hospital to train as a nurse.

In 1887 Florence Nightingale had lamented the fact that young women from the lower middle classes were not becoming nurses. 'We have not yet succeeded in enlisting the better sort of women of tradesmen's families, who generally lead the most useless and uninteresting lives,' she wrote. 'Tradeswomen might lead such good, active lives, like ladies, if they saw the way.' So she would have approved of Alice, the daughter of a coal merchant and the best sort of girl – positive, caring and hard-working – committing herself to a proper two-year, hospital-based course in nursing.

The public image of the profession was wonderfully feminine, and a girl could have a romantic view of her vocation, which did not threaten her ambition to be a wife. An early article for young women considering nursing put the point strongly:

> here is an opportunity for showing how a woman's work may complement the man's in the true order of nature. Where does the character of 'helpmeet' come out so strikingly as in the sick-room, where the quick eye, the soft hand, the light step, and the ready ear, second the wisdom of the physician, and execute his behests better than he himself could have imagined?

In the large general hospitals the nurses were organized on class lines, and the upper- or middle-class girls who became sisters and matrons were in a unique position to demonstrate that, soft hands and light steps at the ready, they would make brilliant wives for the young doctors who had little social life outside the hospital. The rules stated that there was to be no fraternization between nurses and doctors, but they were rarely followed, and marriage kept the turnover of nurses very high. Sadly, Alice was not well placed to find a doctor husband: her hospital was too small and her social class too low.

The backbreaking reality of Alice's job was at odds with images of the nurse as a soft and feminine assistant to her doctor colleagues. A 1909 manual called *How to Become a Nurse* urged young ladies considering a hospital training to have no illusions about the work involved. Before signing up, it recommended: 'place yourself for a month or two under the orders of your own housemaid (if she is a thoroughly trained servant) and let her show you how to clean a room, dust, sweep, clean out grates, clean silver, lay the cloth, light fires etc. . . . a good deal of manual work falls to the lot of probationer'. Domestic service, however, was not considered a good preparation for nursing, 'not because it is not an honourable calling, but because it includes many who have acquired an unsatisfactory tone and demeanour'. The working classes, the manual implied, had the physical but not the mental qualities required.

Even middle-class girls, with their superior outlook on life, should prepare themselves psychologically for the ordeal ahead. *How to Become a Nurse* told them to

> concentrate your efforts on bringing help and cheer to those of your own household, and discipline your mind by turning it courageously away from painful and morbid thoughts. If you aspire to be a source of strength to sick people, you must know how to govern your own thoughts and banish such as sap your energy and faith.

The manual sold well, was updated yearly, and was hugely informative for girls like Alice. At a general hospital, it explained, probationers

> get up at half past six, have breakfast, say prayers. Wash up the breakfast things, clean lamps, spatulas etc., dust the ward, scrub lockers and doctors' tables, wash window sills, serve the patients' lunch, clear and wash up the luncheon things, help nurse with the patients when required, assist with the patients' dinner.

The afternoon brought more waitressing, along with cleaning of the urine glasses and spitting-cups, and making up the fires for the night. The day drew to a close at half past nine with more prayers. After that, girls were to go to their rooms, and had an hour or so free time until the gas was put out at quarter past eleven.

There was stiff competition for in-hospital training, which was open only to women between the ages of 20 and 30. Younger girls were considered too immature, and 'the entire subordination required of the probationer is less easy for older women to accept with good grace'. Alice did well to gain a place at the tiny Hitchin hospital, which had only 26 beds and a nursing staff of one matron, two nurses and three probationers. The entry qualification was 'evidence of character, education, health and physique', and a £10 fee was to be paid for a place on the course. In return laundry and an indoor uniform were provided, and a separate bedroom for each nurse. On completion of her training, Alice's job prospects were good. The number of nursing jobs was increasing rapidly – the 1851 census had recorded only 7,619 patients in hospitals in England and Wales, but by 1901 the number had risen to 39,184. And professionally trained nurses were particularly well placed to find jobs, since they were in the minority.

Nursing paid less than teaching but carried the extra status associated with the saintliness of ministering to the sick, and it gave a woman a proper role in the functioning of the nation. In February 1909 the *Nursing Times* urged its readers to join at once a 'Territorial Force' of nurses trained to deal with wartime situations, suggesting that they go and see 'the patriotic play of which all London is speaking'. This was *The Englishman's Home*, at Wyndham's Theatre, which came as 'a revelation to a somewhat phlegmatic public' in its presention of a Britain vulnerable to attack by foreign forces. (The plot involved a plucky and courageous Mr Brown being shot dead after defending his home, 'Myrtle Villas', against invaders of no fixed nationality but vaguely Prussian.) The next month, the *Nursing Times* carried a follow-up article on the treatment of gunshot wounds. So the natural alliance of nurses and soldiers was in the air.

On completing her training, Alice moved to Southsea, the seaside resort to the east of Portsmouth Harbour, and took a job nursing an elderly man, Mr Holt – a 'confirmed invalid'. Work in a private house was a more attractive option than nursing in a hospital. In general, the hours were shorter and the tasks less strenuous; there was no matron to tyrannize you, and the pay was better. There were plenty of private situations to choose from, since anyone who could afford it preferred to be nursed at home, partly because it was still believed, with some justification, that a hospital stay led inexorably to a hospital death. The rich 'entered the hospitals only to visit, inspect or govern', and more nurses worked in private households than in hospitals.

The 1911 census shows Alice to be boarding at Beach Mansions on St Helen's Parade, Southsea. The enormous mansion block sits at the edge of reclaimed marshland facing out to the Solent and the Isle of Wight – a lovely location on a hot summer's day when Southsea would be busy with holidaymakers, but exposed and windswept in the bitter cold of winter. Twenty-one people were living at her address, many of them the young domestic servants who looked after the boarders and the summer visitors.

Among them were Violet, the pantry maid, Emily the parlour maid, Lilian the housemaid, Alice the sewing maid, Nellie Gratwick the kitchen maid and Nellie Taylor the 'between maid'. The other boarders were older – there was James Sutherland the retired army officer, James Hickman the retired army surgeon, Henry the lighterman, and George the retired inspector of machinery. Alice, then aged 23, gives her profession as 'sick-nurse'. She is the youngest of the boarders, the only single woman amongst them, and the only working woman.

Alice kept her job with Mr Holt, a retired banker, for three years, and managed to save up £60 – a year's salary for a domestic nurse, and nearly two years' salary for a hospital nurse. Being a sensible young woman, she sent the money home for her father to look after. A few years earlier, Charles Burnham had passed on his coal business to Alice's brother Norman and taken up fruit-growing. At the same time, he had given his three daughters a gift of £40 each. He had, at Alice's request, held on to her money – so was now safeguarding a full £100 for her.

By 1913, Alice's life in Southsea was well established, safe and secure. On the negative side, though, she was cut off from her family, and able to make only occasional trips home. And in March 1913 she suffered a shock when her doctor, Bertram Stone, told her that she had peritonitis – a life-threatening inflammation of the bowel linings – and needed a 'somewhat severe abdominal operation'. The surgery was a success. 'She bore the anaesthetic well,' said Dr Stone later. He thought that, despite her plumpness, her heart must have been 'quite sound' and that her general health was good. Indeed, he thought her 'a strong, healthy, robust girl.'

In mid-September Alice's love life suddenly blossomed. She met an older man who, despite being 40, was still single. His looks were reasonable enough – he was slim and well turned out, much taller than her and physically fit. His dark-brown hair was flecked with grey, his complexion was on the pale side and his features were rather thin, but he wasn't, by any reckoning, ugly. He was a man of the world, with a good line in conversation, and he was so well-off, he told her, that he did not need to work. Most significantly, though, he seemed utterly bewitched by Alice, and intent on courting her. His name was George Smith, and he was renting rooms at 80 Kimberley Road, Southsea.

We know very little of what happened between George and Alice during the following weeks – only that Alice came to have tea with her admirer in his rooms at Kimberley Road, and that a month after meeting him, she wrote to her family saying that she intended to marry. She had met George, she wrote, at the Congregationalist Chapel in Southsea. Maybe that was true, or perhaps she was telling a mild lie in order to make them think well of him. Either way, she presented him as a good religious man, and suggested that she bring him home on a visit as soon as possible.

A surviving letter from George Smith to Alice's mother Elizabeth, dated 22 October 1913, gives a sense of the correspondence that had recently passed back and forth between Southsea and Aston Clinton. 'I was pleased with the purport of your letters to Alice,' writes George, somewhat pompously.

> I am now looking forward to coming to Aston Clinton to see you all. You mentioned in your last letter whether we quite understood each other, my answer to that question is yes, and what is more, we love each other. I have never given it a thought as to whether I should be comfortable during my stay at your home, but I could make myself happy anywhere so long as Alice was with me. I have also travelled a great deal and can adapt myself to circumstances.

And he told Mrs Burnham that he and Alice would be leaving Willesden Junction on the 3.13 train the following Saturday, and would bring only a small bag with them.

Charles Burnham met the couple at Tring station in his pony-trap, and took them to see Alice's brother Norman and sister Elizabeth, who both lived nearby. 'They talked to us about marriage,' said Norman, 'and he said he had money. He said he had never done any work and did not intend to do any.' When they arrived at 'Yew Trees', the home of Alice's parents, George continued to boast that he was a man of independent means; he also presented himself as a Congregationalist and talked about religion – but 'refused to give any account of himself except that he had been in Canada where he owned some land; that he was born in Kensington and his father was a drinking man'. In all, the impression that George made on the Burnhams, and in particular on Charles, was very bad. The physical description they gave of him was deeply negative. He had a somewhat pointed chin, they said, a wrinkled neck, and he walked in a stiff-kneed fashion, with his toes pointing outward. And there was something spivvish about his manner. He smoked cigarettes, dressed with a bow tie, wore a gold ring, and carried a watch with illuminated numerals and hands, with a large seal attached to its chain.

On Wednesday, 29 October, Charles Burnham drove George and Alice to Toddington in Bedfordshire, to see Alice's sister Annie, who had married in the summer of 1912. Alice had given her a wedding gift of £10, but Annie had been reluctant to accept such a generous present and had insisted on giving Alice an IOU in case she ever wanted the money back. When Annie later spoke of George and Alice's visit, two aspects seem to have stuck in her mind – George's presentation of himself as a man who did not need to earn his living, and Alice's wish to talk privately about the £10 IOU. The following day, Thursday, the visitors returned to Aston Clinton. George and Alice had intended to stay for several more days, but by now Charles Burnham's distrust of his daughter's fiancé had festered and rooted, and become a deep loathing. He did not wish the marriage to take place, and did not want the man staying in his house any longer. And when, without his consent, George and Alice gave notice of their intended marriage at the church in Aston Clinton, he was distraught. Charles Burnham would later claim that he sensed that George was evil. Indeed, he thought him so bad that he feared 'something serious would happen', and said that he could not sleep while George was under his roof. Whatever he thought at the time, he was sufficiently alienated from his prospective son-in-law to tell Alice that she had better cut her visit short and take George Smith away.

In the circumstances cheerful, sunny, sensible Alice might have been expected to have second thoughts about her wedding. She had always been close to her family, and their opinion on such a momentous event in her life must have been of great importance to her. But she did not give way to her father's judgement, or his authority. She did not take time out to weigh up his fears about George's character. Instead, with no hesitation, she left Aston Clinton on Friday and returned to Southsea with George. By Sunday she had left Beach Mansions and moved into his lodgings at 80 Kimberley Road, taking a separate rented room.

The following Monday she and George went to see Charles Pleasance, a local insurance agent, who already knew George. A few weeks earlier he had turned up at Mr Pleasance's office and had invested a huge sum of money – £1,300 – in an annuity. He now explained that his friend, Miss Burnham, wished to purchase an insurance policy on her life, ensuring a payout of £1,000 if she died. Mr Pleasance asked why she wished to take out the policy, and it was George who answered. 'My friend . . . is the daughter of a well-to-do landed people in Hertfordshire,' he said, 'and is contemplating marriage.' 'Miss Burnham said very little,' said Mr Pleasance, 'and seemed to agree with what Smith had said.' George Smith didn't mention that he was Alice's intended husband. Within hours of her visit to Mr Pleasance, Alice handed in her notice to the 'confirmed invalid', Mr Holt.

The next day, Tuesday, 4 November, she and George were married at the local register office.

Alice's wedding day was not the stuff of fairy tales. That evening, at about 7.30, she was not celebrating with friends or drinking champagne. Instead, she and George paid a visit to Dr Harold Burrows, a Southsea doctor who worked for the North British and Mercantile Insurance Company, and who had been asked to examine her with a view to the company insuring her life. Alice introduced George to Dr Burrows not as her husband but as her fiancé. 'I examined her, and found her sound. I examined her heart and found it quite healthy,' said the doctor. Another task assigned for her wedding day was to write to her father. She told Charles Burnham that she was now married, and asked him to send on the £100 that he had been looking after for her. He received the letter the following morning and, consumed by suspicion and hostility, resolved to hang on to the money.

But Charles Burnham's stubbornness in withholding Alice's savings was easily matched by George Smith's determination to get hold of them. On 11 November he wrote to his father-in-law:

> Sir,
>
> The views and actions which you have been pleased to take towards our marriage are both inconsistant and contemptable – you absolutely appear to be quite out of touch with the methods and principals by which every day life is handled . . . Moreover having failed in your attempt to wreck all possibilities of marriage you take shelter in obdurateness, contempt and remorse . . . What earthly right have you to scorn your daughter in these ways? Is the record of your family so full of virtue that you dispise and grudge your daughter's bright prospects? . . . I remind you that by causing friction broadcast as you have is the greatest mistake of your life time. It is mentioned in the letter Alice received on the 11th inst that as I have an income – the £100

and interest should stand over. A more foolish and elegal action I have never heard – the money is payable on demand, failing which I will take the matter up myself without delay.

He signed himself G. Smith.

Charles Burnham was a respected man, a trusted coal merchant and conscientious fruit farmer. And he was a pillar of the church. What was he to make of such vulgarity and greed? Of such illiteracy, ignorance and aggression? At a loss, he took himself off to Somerset House in London, where the records were kept of the nation's births and marriages, in search of the origins of George Joseph Smith, born in Kensington. But his trip was fruitful only in its confirmation of his misgivings – he found no trace of the man. Charles Burnham also consulted his solicitor. Given his suspicions about George, he wondered, could he legally withhold Alice's money? The question became more pertinent when, on 18 November, George wrote once more to Charles threatening legal action if the money were not surrendered before the 23rd. On the 22nd Alice sent a letter to her father.

> It is a pity that the only path left open to me is to go with my husband to see a solicitor and make a claim upon my father, but before doing so I will wait till the first post Tues. 25th inst. I regret to say this is the last application I can make before going to law. I am very sorry you should have treated my husband and myself in the way you have and I cannot account for such an unjust treatment and it hurts.

She signed off in a voice that sounded more her own: 'I hope you and mother are well Dad.'

On the same day, Charles' solicitor sent a letter designed to buy a little time.

> We need hardly say that if she desires her father to send this money it will be forwarded in due course. It is not unnatural that Mr Burnham should be concerned that his daughter should have married a man about whom he knows so little,

and he desires us to ask you to be good enough to forward to us particulars of the date and place of your birth, and information as to the names, position and place of abode of your parents.

Of course, this was quite different from the letter that George was hoping to receive, and he dashed off a postcard to Charles, spewing bile and sarcasm:

Sir,
In answer to your application regarding my parentage etc. My mother was a Buss Horse, my Father a Cab Driver, my sister a rough rider over the Artic Regions. My Brothers were all gallant sailors on a Steam roller . . . Your despised son-in-law,
G. Smith

His card was accompanied by a letter from Alice, saying simply that she had, that morning, instructed her solicitor to 'take extreme measures' to obtain her money. Three days later George sent another postcard to Charles. 'I do not know your next move', he wrote. 'But take my advice and be very careful.'

The Burnhams' determination to stand up to George now seemed broken. He had also sent unpleasant letters to Alice's sister Annie demanding that she send on the £10 that Alice had given Annie for her wedding. In these he threatened legal action and wrote: 'one has only to look at your face to see what a character you are'. On 25 November Annie dispatched the £10 to Southsea, taking care to pay extra at the post office to obtain a receipt. She was mortified at Alice's collusion in her husband's brutish acts. 'I could not understand,' she said, 'how it was she turned against us after she met her husband.'

Alice's father, Charles, now realized that he had no choice but to release her £100 savings, though it clearly broke his heart to do so – and he sent off the money. At the same time he took the precaution of contacting the police and asking them to make enquiries in Southsea. Detective Constable Stewart Williams of

Portsmouth Borough Constabulary undertook the task of 'ascertaining whether Smith was a man of substance or an adventurer'. Some time in early December he called at 80 Kimberley Road, where Alice and George were still living. The couple were out, so he spoke to the landlady, Annie Page, who told him that Smith seemed to be 'a straightforward man' and that he paid his way. The constable returned another day, when George and Alice were at home. 'I saw him in the sitting-room with his wife,' he said. 'I asked him for his credentials. He said he was independent and demanded to know why I was enquiring.' George told DC Williams that he knew that Alice's father was behind the visit, and he showed the policeman his bank passbook, to demonstrate his much-vaunted financial status. Overall, Stewart Williams concluded that George Smith was 'a man of suspicious appearance'. Alice, by contrast, was a woman 'of a superior kind'. He noted that 'she seemed frightened to speak'.

In late November George revealed to the Southsea insurance agent Charles Pleasance that he had married Alice. That would mean, explained Mr Pleasance, that Alice would need to pay a married woman's premium on her life insurance policy. George was unwilling to pay the premium – and instead reduced the £1,000 policy to £500. That being agreed, Alice paid the first instalment.

At some time during the insurance negotiations George was alone with Charles Pleasance and told him, 'Now I am married I think I ought to make a will leaving everything to my wife, as a married man should do.' The agent advised him to see a solicitor, and George replied: 'I prefer not to have anything to do with solicitors.' So Charles Pleasance drafted him a quick specimen will, leaving everything to Alice which, at George's request, was signed and witnessed by the insurance agent and one of his clerks. 'I think this will do as it is,' George stated, though Mr Pleasance appeared none too sure. George also told the insurance agent that he 'would never think of allowing his wife to make one'. But the fact was that Alice, alone, visited a solicitor's office in Portsmouth at eleven in the morning of 8 December and asked to make a will leaving all she had to her husband. The will, being simple, took only a short time to draw up, and at about noon the same day, she signed it.

George now suggested that he take Alice away on honeymoon to Blackpool – the seaside capital of the north. On leaving Southsea, George told the landlady, Annie Page, that he and Alice would be away for about a week, and suggested that, if she could, she should rent the room out in that time.

They arrived in Blackpool in the descending darkness of a December afternoon, and began the search for a room. Susannah Marsden, a widow who ran a boarding-house in Adefield Street, remembered a couple from Portsmouth coming to the front door. 'I showed them a room on the first floor,' she said, 'and they agreed to take it, but after some conversation the man said: "Is there a Bathroom?" I said "No." He then said, "Well, this won't do for us if there is no Bathroom."' So Mrs Marsden recommended that they try nearby Regent Road, where she knew that the boarding-houses had bathrooms. 'They were in my house only five minutes,' she said. 'I had no conversation with the woman. She was present the whole of the time, but asked no questions.'

The landlady at 16 Regent Road was also a widow. Margaret Crossley lived there with her daughter, Alice, and son-in-law, Joseph (who also had the surname Crossley), and her granddaughter, Maggie. Margaret Crossley answered the knock on the front door at about 5 p.m. George asked whether she had a combined bed-sitting-room to let, and when she said that, yes, she did, it was Alice who asked 'Have you a bath?' When it became clear that Margaret Crossley was able to offer a bathroom, George replied, 'That's all right then,' and the two came into the house. 'Can we have tea?' George asked. 'Yes, what would you like, and at what time?' said Mrs Crossley. George requested 'a plain tea at 6 o'clock', and the couple went up to the bed-sitting-room on the first floor, followed by the landlady and her daughter, Alice. They saw the room and 'appeared satisfied,' said Mrs Crossley. 'I went downstairs and left my daughter with them to prepare the room. Shortly afterwards they left the house saying they were going to fetch the luggage.' They returned at about 6 p.m. with a reddish-brown hold-all. 'They had some tea and did some writing,' said Mrs Crossley. 'Smith asked me what time the post went out and I said, "at 8 o'clock if you want to be in time for stamps".' They went out at 7.30 and returned at ten and went to bed. Mrs Crossley saw no more of them that night. She did, though, notice that Alice appeared to be in good health, 'and was very cheerful.'

At about 8 o'clock the following morning the bell from the first-floor sitting-room rang, and Margaret Crossley's daughter went up to see what was wanted by the guests. When she arrived, she found that George had gone out already and that Alice wished her to tidy the room. She 'bade me Good Morning', said Alice Crossley, 'and said, "I had a splendid night's rest, the best night I have had for a long time."' Shortly afterwards, George Smith returned and the couple had their breakfast. Sometime just before 10 a.m. Margaret Crossley found her guests in the lobby and took the opportunity to ask if they would be wanting dinner. George offered to go out and buy food, and Mrs Crossley told him that she could provide vegetables and pudding. So George ordered potatoes, and said he and Alice would buy some chops. 'While talking about dinner, I enquired if they had slept all right, and were comfortable', said Mrs Crossley. Alice had replied: 'Yes, with the exception of a slight headache through travelling, otherwise I had a good night.' Then they left the house.

Margaret Crossley saw the Smiths several times that day. They returned during the morning with their chops, then again at

1 p.m. for dinner. They spent the afternoon in town, and finished off their afternoon's entertainments with a visit to a local doctor – George Billing. George Smith introduced the doctor to Alice, and explained that she had 'a headache and maziness owing to a long journey'. Alice did not seem at all distressed by her headache, in fact the doctor described her as 'quite cheerful', though he also thought her 'rather tired'. 'She was a short, pale woman, extremely fat,' he said. But 'from a medical point of view she looked quite healthy'. Her pulse might have been slightly slow, he remembered later, but 'nothing out of the way.' He asked about the state of her bowels, and learned that she was constipated; he also examined her tongue, which was coated. He prescribed some headache pills 'made of acetanilide, caffeine and heroin,' which, he said, 'relieves the headache through the blood system.' He kept these pills ready-made at his surgery, and gave her a small box containing a dozen. And he gave her a 'stomach mixture' made up from bicarbonate of soda, rhubarb, gentian and chloroform water. His fee was 3s 6d, which George paid immediately.

The couple then returned to 16 Regent Road with 'a small quantity of butter and a small tin of milk', in time for their tea, which was once more made by Alice Crossley. Alice's headache was, apparently, sufficiently disturbing for her to mention it in a postcard which she posted that day to her sister Elizabeth. But, by the evening, it was not bad enough to stop her visiting the cinema.

Friday, 12 December was the third day of George and Alice's honeymoon, and began with a hearty breakfast of bacon, which they had bought and the Crossleys had cooked and taken up to the bed-sitting-room on the first floor. At about 10 a.m. they came downstairs, and Margaret Crossley asked after Alice and her headache. It wasn't better, she said, and she wished it would 'clear away'. Still, it didn't prevent her from accompanying George on an excursion to buy stewing steak for dinner. Would they like pudding? Mrs Crossley asked when they returned – and George replied, yes they would like tapioca. The schedule for the day was much the same as before. They had dinner at 1 p.m. and went into town afterwards, returning at 5 o'clock for toast and tea. At 6.15 that evening Margaret Crossley went up to the bed-sitting-room to clear up after the meal, and found that Alice was at the table, writing a postcard. George, said Mrs Crossley, 'was standing behind her looking over her shoulder. He pointed to something she had written and said "I shouldn't put that."' Shortly afterwards Alice and George went out to catch the post. Before she left, Alice went down to the kitchen and asked Alice Crossley to prepare a hot bath, which she would take when she got back.

The card that Mrs Burnham received the next day was post-marked 7.15 p.m., 12 December 1913. It read:

My dear Mother,

We arrived here last Wednesday, have very nice comfortable apartments and find Blackpool a lovely place. I am sorry to say I have again suffered with bad headaches and which necessitated my seeing a doctor – am taking medicine. My husband does all he possibly can for me – in fact dear, I have the best husband in the world. With fond love from us both.

Yrs lovingly,

Alice

xxxxx

She had also, during the stay, sent two postcards to her sister Elizabeth. The first said she had just arrived, but had a headache. The second, said Elizabeth, mentioned the headache again, and said 'that her husband had insisted on her seeing a Doctor, and that he had done all he could for her.'

When George and Alice returned to the house just before 8 o'clock, Alice Crossley went to prepare the bathroom, which was on the same floor as the Smiths' bed-sitting-room. The bedroom was at the front of the house and the bathroom at the back – separated only by a carpeted landing and three steps. Alice Crossley lit the gas lights and pulled the blind on the window down, but left it to Alice to run the water, since the bath was plumbed in and had taps. Shortly afterwards, Alice Crossley had finished her work and was about to return to her mother in the kitchen when she saw Alice Smith going towards the bathroom. She asked her not to put too much hot water in, 'as the water was not too hot.' Alice replied: 'All right. Goodnight.' Sound travelled easily in the house, and Margaret Crossley overheard her daughter give the instruction about the water.

While Alice took her bath, Margaret, Alice and Joseph Crossley were in the kitchen, which was directly beneath the bathroom. At about a quarter past eight Margaret Crossley noticed water seeping through the ceiling and running down the walls of the kitchen. Joseph Crossley also noticed a drop of water fall from the ceiling. 'That lady must have filled the bath too full,' he said to his wife, 'You should go and tell her about it.' But Alice Crossley thought it best not to interfere. 'No,' she said. 'She might have splashed a little drop over, she will think that I am complaining about it. I will tell her next time.' Joseph Crossley then left the house to go to his work at the Clifton Hotel. Margaret Crossley's version of the same conversation was that she had said, 'Oh Alice, go and tell Mrs Smith not to fill the bath,' and her daughter's reply had been, 'Oh, Mother, they will think we are grumbling. Do not let us say anything now.'

About ten minutes after the family had noticed the dripping water, George Smith came downstairs and appeared in the kitchen, bringing with him two eggs. He handed them to Margaret Crossley, saying that he and Alice would like them for breakfast the following morning. Mrs Crossley took the eggs, and George stayed in the kitchen, chatting for about ten minutes. He had learned that a new motor fire engine was going to be tested in Blackpool on Monday, he said, and he thought he would go and see it. Much later, when she looked back on it, Mrs Crossley said: 'I wondered what was the matter with him, he looked so wild and agitated.'

George then left the kitchen, and Margaret Crossley heard him calling out, 'Alice, when you have done, put the light out.' Thinking that he was calling for Alice Crossley, Margaret sent her daughter to find out what he wanted. She went to the bottom of the stairs, and asked if she were needed. 'No,' said George, 'I was speaking to my wife to put the light out in the bathroom.' Alice Crossley returned to the kitchen and after a few moments, she said: 'I heard him call out "my wife cannot speak to me",' so she returned to the stairs. George Smith was at the top, calling out: 'Go for a doctor, fetch a doctor, fetch Dr Billing, she knows him.'

'Dr Billing lives quite near to my house,' said Margaret Crossley. 'I ran for him, and he came to the house in a few minutes. I waited on the stairs.'

'I went straight up to the bathroom,' said George Billing. There he found George by the side of the bath, holding Alice. She was still in the bath, but positioned the wrong way round with her head at the tap-end. She was raised up by George, in a sort of sitting position, and he was supporting her head with his left arm. 'I did not notice anything particular about his dress,' said Dr Billing, 'except that he had one sleeve of his coat rolled up. I believe it was the left one – the one he was supporting her with.' The water, he noticed, was soapy, and 'came above the breasts,' filling the bath to within an inch of the top.

'Why haven't you lifted her out?' Dr Billing asked George – who replied that he couldn't lift her. Billing then said, 'Why didn't you pull the plug and let the water off?' George replied that he had not thought of it. Together George and Dr Billing lifted Alice out of the bath and laid her on the floor. 'I pumped her,' said Dr Billing, 'but did not get anything, only a mouthful of froth and water.' It did not take him long to realize that she was dead.

Margaret Crossley's granddaughter Maggie had been dispatched to bring Joseph back to the house, and it was he who accompanied Police Sergeant Robert Valiant to a single bedroom on the first floor, where Alice was now lying, covered over with a sheet. 'I examined the body and found no marks of violence,' he said. Taken together, the facts – a plump woman in a bath, no signs of a struggle and other people around in the house – suggested that a horrible accident had occurred. The policeman inspected the bathroom. He noticed that the floor was wet and that there was no clothing lying around. He then went downstairs and told George Smith that he would have to make a statement. Joseph Crossley, George Smith and Robert Valiant walked together to Blackpool police station.

George's statement mentioned Alice's headaches, and stated that after their evening walk Alice had said she wanted a bath.

> About fifteen minutes after she had gone into the bath I called out to her to mind and turn the lights out after you are finished. I got no answer from her, at the same time Mrs Crossley came upstairs thinking I was calling out to her, we both looked into the bathroom and found her under the water. I lifted her head out of the water and held it until the Doctor came, then we lifted her out of the bath. The Doctor examined her and pronounced life extinct.

As George Smith and Joseph Crossley were leaving the police station, a police constable asked George: 'are you going to take her home to bury her or are you going to bury her here?' George replied: 'I will bury her here, I don't see what good it is taking her home as my means are limited.' Robert Valiant witnessed the exchange. Years later, he said he thought George 'very callous and in no way distressed.'

That evening, after Alice's death, George wrote another postcard to her mother. 'Alice is very ill,' it said, 'I will wire you tomorrow.' Maggie Crossley was sent to the post office to post the card. During the commotion, the Crossleys' next-door neighbours, William and Sarah Haynes, had come into the house to help out. William Haynes had helped to lift Alice's body from the bathroom to the bedroom, then went downstairs to join the others in the house. George, he remembered, said to him: 'I would not be surprised at anything after this.' He then left and went upstairs. Margaret Crossley told William Haynes to go after him. George 'went into his room,' said William Haynes, 'and I followed him and saw him take three or four rings off the mantelpiece, which he placed in his purse, making some remarks to the effect that they were her rings. He asked me to have some whisky, which I accepted. Mrs Smith had no rings on her fingers when I carried her to the bedroom.'

Sarah Haynes assisted in laying-out Alice's body, and noticed that 'she had no rings on her fingers.' She also helped clean the bath, and noticed a quantity of 'lady's dark hair adhering to the sides of the broad end of the bath.' When Alice had been found dead, her feet were at the broad end of the bath, and her head at the narrow tap-end. All this struck Sarah Haynes as odd.

> When Mrs Smith was carried out of the bathroom her hair was hanging down loosely, but there were several hairpins in her hair as if she had gone for a bath with her hair pinned up. I have frequently cleaned baths after ladies have bathed, but I have never seen so much hair in a bath as there was on this occasion.

The implication was that Alice had not been intending to get her hair wet. Somehow, though, her head had been under the water at both ends of the bath.

That same evening a local undertaker, John Hargreaves, arrived at 16 Regent Road. George Smith, said John Hargreaves, 'wanted me to bury her and make as cheap a coffin as possible and have her buried in a Public Grave.' Joseph Crossley was listening to the discussion, and objected, saying there should be a good coffin and that if George would not pay, then he would. George's response is not recorded, but, said the undertaker, he 'intimated to me that he wanted the body buried as soon as possible as he wanted to get away as soon as he could.' Margaret Crossley later claimed that as bedtime approached she said to George: 'What are you going to do about sleeping because I won't have you in this house.' George answered: 'Oh I could sleep in the room where she is, she won't hurt me.' But Mrs Crossley insisted that he sleep somewhere else. So he moved in next door, with William and Sarah Haynes.

John Hargreaves returned the following morning to give George some prices for the coffin and burial. George 'said he had not a lot of money to throw away. He said he would have the cheapest as it did not matter to the dead and he would not come to Blackpool any more and it did not matter to him what sort of grave she was buried in.' He ordered a deal coffin, and arranged to have her buried in a public grave. Margaret Crossley asked if Alice's relatives would be coming. George replied: 'No they are too common and too poor.'

That same morning, Saturday, 13 December, George sent a telegram to the Burnhams. It was handed in at Blackpool at 11.30 a.m., and reached Aston Clinton just after midday. It read: 'Alice died last night in her bath, letter following', and was signed 'Smith, 16 Regent Road, Blackpool'. Alice's mother Elizabeth and her brother Norman left that afternoon for Blackpool. They got as far as Preston and stayed there the night. Alice's father Charles remained at home and received the letter from George that followed the telegram. It went through, once more, the phenomenon of Alice's headaches, her trip to the doctor, her request for a bath, and her sudden death. 'I went to the Police Station,' wrote George, 'and asked them to send an Official to come to the house and take particulars which they did. This is

the greatest and most cruel shock that ever a man could have suffered, words cannot describe my feelings. We were so happy
together which she has told all her friends in her letters to them.'
He added that 'the inquest will be held next week', and asked for
details to be sent on relating to Alice's childhood illnesses.

He was lying about the inquest. It was actually held on the same
day that he was writing the letter – the day that Alice died, when
Elizabeth and Norman Burnham were in transit, on their way to
Blackpool. It took place at Blackpool's Central Police Office at
6 p.m., a hundred yards from the Crossley house, where Alice's
body still lay.

Evidence was heard from George, whose touching observation,
'we had only been married six weeks', was recorded in the minutes.
Margaret Crossley spoke, as did Sergeant Robert Valiant and Dr
Billing, who had conducted a post-mortem earlier in the day. He
found no marks on Alice's body, other than the abdominal scar
from the operation that she had recovered from so well earlier in
the year. 'She was a well-nourished woman, very fat,' he said.
Internally, he found that 'the heart was enlarged and the valves dis-
eased as if she had had some rheumatic fever or inflammation round
the valves of her heart. The lungs were full of froth and water and
crackled', showing that she had drowned. The jury's verdict was
that Alice had died accidentally. She had suffered from heart disease, they decided, and had drowned in a hot bath 'probably
through being seized with a fit or a faint'.

After his wife's death, George continued to sleep next door at the
house of William and Sarah Haynes. But Alice Crossley remembered that on Sunday, 14 December, the morning after the
inquest, he was in the downstairs room at 16 Regent Road. Alice
looked out of the window.

I said to him, 'There are some people coming down the street
in black, I wonder if they are looking for you.' He said, 'No

they are not for me, I have got nobody to come.' They came to the house . . . He got up and looked out of the window and said: 'Oh my God, it's her mother and brother. I wish it had been the old man.'

Elizabeth Burnham said later that she and Norman arrived at 16 Regent Road at about 10 a.m. that Sunday. George opened the door, and greeted them with the words: 'I said you wouldn't come, why didn't you drop me a card?' Elizabeth Burnham replied, 'There was no time for that, George.' Norman remembered George speaking about the inquest, and saying that Alice had died from heart failure. He also explained that he had arranged for a funeral the next day, Monday. 'I asked where my sister was,' said Norman, 'and Smith said, "In the Mortuary." Mother said, "Haven't you been to see her?" He said, "No I haven't." She said, "Won't you go with us?" He said, "I'll go if you are going".' So the three of them went off together to see Alice's body. George, Norman remembered, was not in mourning clothes, but wore a black tie. He did not appear very upset and said, 'I have done everything I could and my conscience is clear.' They all then had dinner at the Crossleys. During the afternoon, George played the piano.

He also, at some point, dashed out to the undertaker's office. John Hargreaves remembered him calling in and asking if his earlier request for a public grave could now be altered. 'He said his wife's mother and brother had come unexpectedly and he did not want them to know that he was burying her in a public grave.' Mr Hargreaves explained that he could not arrange a private grave in time for the next day but would be able to do it if the funeral were delayed by one day, until Tuesday. George, however, was adamant that the funeral should take place as soon as possible. So it was to be a common grave after all.

On Monday, 15 December, John Hargreaves took the coffin to the mortuary and placed Alice's body in it. 'I screwed her down shortly before [the funeral],' he said. It was Hargreaves who put the coffin on a hand-trolley and pulled it to the chapel in the local cemetery. After a short service, the coffin was trundled along to the grave. The few mourners had arrived at the cemetery by tramcar – just George, Alice's mother and her brother, and the Crossleys. George, Alice Crossley remembered, 'had no black clothes and did not get any with the exception of a black tie which my mother induced him to buy. He wore a heavy green mixture overcoat and a blue peaked cap to the funeral.'

'Owing to the funeral arrangements being made so quickly,' said Norman, 'we were unable to obtain a wreath and Smith hadn't got one, so there were no flowers.' Afterwards, the little group made its way back to Blackpool. Elizabeth Burnham said:

> Smith left us, saying he wanted to catch the 12 o'clock train . . .
> I said to him, 'What are you going to do with Alice's clothes?'
> He said, 'I'll see to it, which of her sisters are most in need.' I
> gave him the address of my two other daughters and he took
> something down . . . He said, 'I will write a nice letter to you
> when I get back.' When he was leaving us I said, 'You will
> write won't you?' He said, 'Yes I will.' This was the last I ever
> saw or heard of him.

4

Art and Science in the Courtroom

BERNARD SPILSBURY'S LIFE in the mortuaries of north-west London was little changed. The jobs that came his way were the usual sad stories of suicide or accidental death – the chloroform cases, the botched home abortions, the undernourished or abandoned infants. It is hard to know what it does to the soul of a man to spend so many hours in the presence of death – exploring and analysing it – but there is something about Spilsbury's case-cards that transcends (or surrenders) clinical detachment. The definition of the word 'autopsy' incorporates this human element, suggesting something beyond purely scientific examination. An autopsy is a 'personal inspection' or 'critical dissection'. It is suggestive of the real relationship between the pathologist and the dead – a duty of care and of justice.

In London, the morgue and the mortuary were private places. In Paris, until 1907, the morgue was public theatre. Emile Zola wrote of it in his fiction:

> There are the regulars who do the rounds so as not to miss one of these shows of death. When the slabs are empty, the people go out disappointed, feeling as if they have been swindled, muttering between their teeth. When the slabs are well-furnished, when there is a good show of human flesh, the visitors flock there to get a cheap thrill. They are scared, they joke or applaud, or hiss as in the theatre, and go away satisfied . . . Amongst them would be found the workshop wag, making his audience smile with a joke about the expression of every corpse; they called the

burnt bodies 'coal merchants'; the hanged, the murdered, the drowned, the bodies pierced with holes or crushed, aroused their bantering humour . . .

The British, deprived of the chance to view the dead at home, visited the morgue in Paris as part of a tourist itinerary that included the Eiffel Tower and the Louvre. By the end of the nineteenth century, the attraction drew around a million people a year.

Spilsbury's experience with the dead was different. It was intensely private. The mortuary was the hidden part of the hospital, and the bodies he investigated had been removed from their usual environment – the place of death, the laying-out, the undertaker. As he cut them open, with the pathologist's routine first long incision down the torso, he entered their world as it was in the final moments of life, searching for clues. In the case of a post-mortem on a nameless male infant in April 1913, he discovers that though the baby, aged between 10 and 12 months, was found dead in a ditch and covered in burns, he was killed not by fire but by rickets and acute bronchitis. He notes that a lock of hair has been cut, and writes: 'No indication of neglect or ill treatment. Attempt to destroy body in fire. In doubled up position.'

The work inside the mortuary was slice-by-slice, observation-by-observation, intensive and focused, and somewhat suited to Spilsbury's introverted character. People found him quiet, serious and painstaking. And his work spilled over into his home life. In 1912 he decided that Harrow was too far away from Paddington, and he moved his family to a large semi-detached house in St John's Wood. His wife, Edith, was pregnant with their second child, and the new house at 31 Marlborough Hill gave them more space. But, equally as important, extra rooms allowed Spilsbury to have a study on the ground floor, and to set up a laboratory in the attic, properly equipped so that he could bring samples home from the hospital and the mortuaries, and carry on working into the night.

There is no record of Edith's reaction to this new development, or to the fact that outside the home laboratory and hospital death-rooms, in the daylight world of police investigations, trials and newspapers, her husband's life was changing. Bernard Spilsbury was on the cusp of becoming a public figure. His performance at the trial of Dr Crippen in 1910 had impressed the authorities, and he was offered the post of official Home Office Pathologist. His St Mary's colleague, William Willcox, was now his immediate superior both at the Home Office and the hospital. His mentor, Augustus Pepper, retired. The shuffling of positions meant that Spilsbury entered the first rank of forensic science and became part of the British establishment – an insider. He undoubtedly enjoyed his new status, but not being a gregarious man, he didn't capitalize on the social side of his elevation. Instead, he used it to dig in professionally. He seemed to relish the fact that, for him, Crippen was a springboard, and made it his business to establish himself as an unimpeachable witness at the big criminal trials that, from time to time, came his way.

He had much to learn. In the post-mortem room he was in control, the boss. But in a courtroom he had to earn his place, establish his authority in the face of cross-examinations by clever lawyers. There was one barrister in particular who with the sheer force of his personality demonstrated how to take control of a trial, like a ringmaster at a circus. He was Edward Marshall Hall: the man who had boasted that, had he represented Dr Crippen, he would have saved him from the gallows. Marshall Hall was the most sought-after defending barrister of his day (his nickname was 'the Great Defender'), while the St Mary's team were invariably the expert witnesses for the Crown. Clashes were inevitable.

Marshall Hall's career was built on theatricality, and it helped that, like Bernard Spilsbury, he was tall and exceptionally handsome. Everyone remarked on it. One friend, the playwright Arthur Pinero, thought him, 'a revelation of manly beauty'. Another, Edward Marjoribanks, said he was 'endowed with pre-eminent personal beauty of the most virile type'. In the opinion of the politician F. E. Smith: 'He was a man of remarkable appearance. Very greatly above the average height, admirably proportioned, exceptionally handsome, he radiated vigour, courage and personality.'

In court, he viewed himself as an actor on a stage. Except, he said, 'I have no scenes to help me, and no words are written for me to say . . . But, out of the vivid, living dream of somebody else's life, I have to create an atmosphere – for that is advocacy.' He liked to throw caution to the wind, to come up with startling theories and images, gesturing dramatically while raising or lowering his voice for added drama. As F. E. Smith observed:

> The élan with which he swept down upon a doubtful jury, brushing aside their prejudices, and persuading them against their will, sometimes possibly against their better judgement, into accepting his own, sanguine view of his client's innocence, won many a day which a more timorous, if not less skilful advocate must have given up for lost.

He seemed entirely unembarrassed by his failure to grasp difficult legal concepts – and instead made a feature of it. In the middle of a trial, he would whisper loudly to his junior, '*You* must take this point, there's some law in it.' But he was far from stupid and was quite capable of tearing apart an ill-prepared or ambiguous expert testimony.

The case which defined him, at which he perfected his style, was a murder trial of 1909 that was held in Wolverhampton but made national news. A local brewer called Edward Lawrence was accused of having shot and killed his lover, Ruth Hadley. Lawrence was known to be violent when drunk, and had recently been convicted for savagely biting a police constable. The prosecution evidence was strong. Lawrence had arrived at the house of his local doctor, flustered and saying that he had shot a woman. The doctor rushed to Lawrence's house and found Ruth Hadley lying on the floor with a gunshot wound to the head and another to the arm. Lawrence was ranting, 'For God's sake do everything you can for her', and then 'I'm glad I did it. She is best dead.'

At the trial, the outlook for Lawrence initially seemed very black. But Marshall Hall conducted the defence with tremendous aplomb. He painted a picture of Ruth Hadley as a wild, jealous and violent woman who was terrified that Lawrence would leave her. He produced a string of witnesses who testified that Ruth had often threatened to shoot Lawrence, and that she had regularly assaulted him – on one occasion with a hat-pin, on another with an umbrella handle. Then he put the defendant himself in the witness-box; and in a cool, considered manner, Lawrence related that both he and Ruth had been drunk on the night of her death. She had thrown crockery and fire-irons at him, and he had gone to his bedroom to fetch his revolver. He had fired wide, to frighten her, but by mistake caught her arm. When he returned to the bedroom to hide the gun, she had followed him upstairs and found it again. Ruth appeared in the dining-room with the weapon, said Lawrence, and pointed it at him. He had gripped her wrist, and in the struggle the gun had gone off, hitting her in the temple. She had dropped to the floor.

Marshall Hall plunged into his final speech. Ruth, he said, 'had taken that revolver down, knowing that her life with Lawrence was finished and intending to finish Lawrence too. She was desperate, defiant, dangerous.' He asked each member of the jury to imagine the scene; and as he did so, he picked up the revolver. 'When he entered the room,' he said, 'he saw her pointing her revolver like this.' And he lunged at the jury with the gun. 'He saw the hammer rising, as you may see it rising now as I pull the trigger . . .' The judge was persuaded. He summed up in favour of the defendant, and the jury took just twenty minutes to reach a verdict of 'not guilty'. It was the ultimate demonstration of the power of Marshall Hall's performance.

By 1912 Edward Marshall Hall was at the top of his game. But just as he peaked, it seemed that the world around him was changing, and that his style was in danger of becoming outmoded. There were elements of the Victorian theatre about Marshall Hall that made him a sort of Henry Irving of the law – a proponent of the grand gesture and extravagant rhetoric. His approach suited the post-Smethurst period in which scientific evidence was out of fashion and ingenious arguments about character and motive could win a case. But in the new century there was a growing sense that science was making a comeback, in general and in the world of the criminal law.

As the Victorian era of trains and telegrams and bridges gave way to a twentieth-century world of motor cars, aeroplanes, submarines, wireless telegraphy and radium, it seemed that a scientific revolution had begun. The change was hard to ignore – motor cars were now a regular feature of the streets, in 1909 Bleriot had crossed the channel by air, and the following year Dr Crippen was caught thanks to Marconi technology. The scientist was the coming man.

Strand Magazine, which published the Sherlock Holmes stories, took a keen interest in the subject, carrying a debate on 'the promise of science' which took seriously the idea that science was a panacea and would soon solve all the ills of the earth. Factories producing cheap and abundant artificial foods were about to take the place of farms, while the farm-free countryside would become a mass of trees and flowers, like a vast garden. An inexhaustible energy supply was, with great confidence, imagined – utilizing heat from deep within the earth. 'This is present everywhere under our feet, and, when turned to account, must inevitably equalise, more or less, the prosperity of all the inhabitants of the globe.' Scientists argued that in this golden age there would be no more wars, because those living in a time of plenty simply would not countenance them.

Some of the experts who participated in the debate dissented from the view that these great benefits would come easily, but most thought that science was transforming the world for the better. Professor E. Ray Lankester predicted other social consequences of the new science. 'Why should lunatics, degenerates and criminals be allowed to marry?' he asked. '[The] science of eugenics has hardly been considered in this country. We know much of the breeding of all animals except man. Why should the moral and physical health of the people not be a matter of prime importance to Government?' The question did not seem out of place or sinister.

The hopes for science in the world of crime were as optimistic as those in agriculture, energy, transport, medicine and everything else. Fingerprints were suddenly all the rage. In 1902 Scotland Yard had set up a fingerprint department, and that year a 41-year-old labourer, Harry Jackson, became the first person to be convicted in the British courts on fingerprint evidence. In 1905 Alfred and Arthur Stratton were tried and hanged on fingerprint evidence for the vicious murder of Thomas and Ann Farrow, and in 1911 Thomas Jennings became the first person in the United States to be convicted, on fingerprint evidence, of murder. *Strand Magazine* carried a piece called 'Fingerprints which have convicted criminals,' filled with information about 'loops, arches, whorls and composites' and enlarged pictures of incriminating prints.

In the thirty years since the confusion over the blood on the knife of Reverend Hayden, science had come a long way. In 1901 Paul Uhlenhuth, a young German bacteriologist, made the discovery that different bloods reacted differently when injected with the blood of another species. Human blood could now be differentiated from animal blood with confidence, and in 1910

Strand Magazine carried an article 'The Detection of Blood Guilt', explaining that the method of identifying human blood was now 'absolutely infallible'.

In January 1908 *Strand Magazine* posed the obvious question: 'Can Criminals be Cured by Surgical Operation?' Dr Bernard Hollander wrote:

> As regards the anatomical marks of the typical criminal, 'we may say at once that there is no "bump" for thieving or murder, but there is a general conformation of the head which characterises the born criminal . . . criminal anthropologists have found that his skull is widest from ear to ear, i.e. [it] is largest in its bi-temporal diameter, and is compressed front to back.'

This may not have been quite the 'exact science' that Arthur Conan Doyle had in mind when he addressed St Mary's Hospital in 1910 – but it was not often easy to distinguish the science that would stand the test of time from that which would not. And Dr Hollander was convinced of his facts:

> It is to the physician that the public will look for the differential diagnosis between the curable and incurable criminal, and it is he who will be largely instrumental in the treatment of moral disease. The surgeon's knife has frequently changed a lunatic to a sane person, there is no reason why it should not change the criminally insane to a moral person.

The confidence in science, and new ambitions for it, were a part of Bernard Spilsbury's working life. He, along with his colleagues Augustus Pepper and William Willcox, had joined a new club – the Medico-Legal Society – at which doctors, lawyers and others with a professional interest regularly debated such subjects. In June 1908 Dr Albert Wilson gave a talk to the Society on 'The Corrective Treatment of the Criminal'. 'I suggest dividing humanity into three groups,' he began. These were, 'the normal, the insane and the degenerate.' The third group, he said, was the most important class 'as he is so hopeless and yet so prolific'. He spoke of his examination of the brain of 'a most degraded man and a murderer'. He had found that the man's brain contained grooves that were 'abnormally shallow', and that a part of it was 'shrivelled'. This, and other cases, had convinced the doctor that 'the degenerate was a victim to bad machinery', and, he concluded, 'must be secluded for the sake of society, as we do with chronic lunatics'. And if he did not respond to treatment by 'firmness, sympathy and emotional religion', then 'we would have to show discretion and courage in a system of painless extinction where such was in the interests of the culprit or of society'.

In the discussion that followed, Earl Russell took the view that 'the criminal classes must be abolished; if punishment will not cure them, they must be secluded, and be prevented from propagating other criminals.' Arnold White agreed that 'it must be seen that the quality of the nation's brain structure was on the increase, otherwise our doom was sealed.' Two doctors, though, were sceptical – thinking that more cases should be studied before making generalizations.

A similarly bracing talk was given in January 1912, this time by Dr Robert Rentoul and titled 'The Prevention of Mental Degeneracy'. He thought there were nearly eight million degenerates in Britain, and that 'degenerates multiply twice as fast as do the sane'. Drastic action was needed, and he urged that all mental degenerates be surgically sterilized. The playwright, George Bernard Shaw, attended the talk and remarked that 'if the principles laid down by Dr Rentoul had been vigorously applied neither he nor Dr Rentoul would have been there.' The doctor's remedy, he thought, impractical at best, since 'whenever we got a degenerate we would have to disable all his brothers and sisters, and his parents, if alive.' Otherwise there was nothing in heredity. Was there anyone present, he asked, 'who had not an insane person or a drunkard in his family'? In the rest of the debate, the speakers were split on the subject, roughly 50 : 50.

In this context, it was no surprise that the public adored a scientific detective like Sherlock Holmes. And when science was touted as the cure for everything from hunger to war, to criminality – the time seemed ripe for the real-life scientific detectives to assert themselves – detectives not to be found in police stations, but in hospital mortuaries. In the years that followed, a number of murder stories hit the headlines that pitted the leading scientific detectives of the day – the St Mary's team – against the paramount practitioner of the law as an art – Edward Marshall Hall. Forensic science was to be interrogated by the sceptical Great Defender, and attacked with unrestrained, unashamed showmanship.

The first such story was the 1912 trial of Frederick Seddon, who was accused of murdering his lodger Eliza Barrow. It was Marshall Hall's first poisoning trial and he trained for it 'like an athlete for a race . . . going to bed early and saturating his mind with works on the scientific questions in the case'. The court heard that Seddon was a hard-working insurance agent from Lancashire, who had an obsession with wealth. Little else seemed to matter to him and he lived to 'turn if possible every transaction of his daily life into a means of making money'. He bragged about money the whole time, and was never embarrassed by the subject. In fact, he 'seemed to be singularly free from the snobbish pursuit of appearance which is so often a weakness of his class'.

In 1909 Seddon had bought a fourteen-room house at 63 Tollington Park in north London, and the following year he decided to gain an income from his home by taking in a lodger. In July 1910 a 49-year-old spinster, Eliza Barrow, moved in with her 10-year-old ward, Ernie Grant. Before long, Seddon had persuaded Miss Barrow to sign over to him a controlling interest in all her savings. In return, he said, he would give her a modest annuity, and allow her to live at Tollington Park rent-free.

In the hot summer of 1911 Eliza Barrow became ill with

agonizing stomach pains. The local doctor, Dr Sworn, prescribed bismuth and morphine, but Miss Barrow grew worse, so Frederick Seddon arranged for her to make a will, of which he was the chief beneficiary. That September Miss Barrow died. The doctor said the death was due to epidemic diarrhoea and exhaustion. An outbreak of diarrhoea was sweeping London – on 17 August *The Times* stated that 548 children had died from it that week. 'There is little doubt also that the infection is largely caused by flies,' the paper reported. The police noted that Frederick Seddon's daughter, Maggie, had been sent out to buy fly-paper in the weeks before Miss Barrow's death. They also observed that fly-papers contained arsenic.

Frederick Seddon arranged Miss Barrow's funeral – taking 12s 6d in commission from the undertaker and ensuring that she was buried in a common grave, although her family had a vault in Islington cemetery. His behaviour made Miss Barrow's relatives suspicious about the circumstances of her death, and on 15 November 1911 her body was exhumed.

Bernard Spilsbury performed the post-mortem at Finchley with William Willcox present. His case-card states that the body of Miss Barrow was 'well nourished'. The skin of the face was brown and mummified, he wrote. But internally, the body was 'extremely well preserved'. Otherwise, there was nothing re-markable to note. He found about 70 calculi, or stones, in the gall-bladder and some 'semi-solid black material' in the stomach. His conclusion was 'no disease to account for death'. The only thing that he noted to be 'consistent with death from gastro enteritis' was the condition of the alimentary canal. The final words on his card are 'No indication of chronic arsenic'.

Both prosecution and defence now focused on the difference between chronic arsenic poisoning, which in all likelihood was accidental, and acute arsenic poisoning – which almost certainly was not. The prosecution took the view that Frederick Seddon had poisoned Miss Barrow with a large dose of arsenic obtained by soaking the fly-paper that Maggie had bought – producing an arsenic-rich liquid that could be added to the 'Valentine's Meat Juice' she liked to take, or to her brandy.

In court, Spilsbury reiterated his opinion that the body 'was very well preserved internally and externally . . . Taking into account that the death took place in September 1911, the state of preservation in which I found the body was very abnormal.' He said that, on internal examination, he did not find the fatty degeneration of the liver or the heart walls that he associated with arsenic poisoning. But, he told the court, 'the preservation of the body was more consistent with acute arsenical poisoning than with epidemic diarrhoea.'

Edward Marshall Hall took the view that if he could show that Miss Barrow suffered from chronic rather than acute arsenic poisoning, then his client would be saved from the hangman. His line, all along, was that Dr Sworn had been right in his judgement that Miss Barrow had died from diarrhoea, but he conceded that the condition might have been aggravated by accidental chronic arsenic poisoning. He cross-examined Spilsbury on the subject, and Spilsbury maintained his position unerringly, acknowledging that people did take small doses of arsenic for medical purposes without ill effect, but reiterating that the highly preserved state of Miss Barrow's body was more consistent with acute poisoning. The young doctor gave clear, concise answers, as he had done in the Crippen case two years earlier, and emerged from Hall's examination unscathed.

However, his senior colleague, William Willcox, suffered a bruising. Willcox had estimated that five grains of arsenic had been administered to Miss Barrow – two grains being a fatal dose. He came to his conclusion by analysing the tiny amounts of arsenic found in various organs of Miss Barrow's body, multiplying them to give an amount (2.01 grains) for the body as a whole, and then multiplying again, to take into account the fact that arsenic is very quickly expelled from the body. Edward Marshall

Hall attacked the whole experiment. It was, he said, flawed. When Willcox calculated the proportions, he had got them wrong: he had forgotten to factor in the different rates of evaporation of water from different body parts. It was a complex point, but it had the effect of making Willcox seem if not incompetent, then fallible. And, of course, it opened up the possibility of science turning out to be unscientific after all. Willcox insisted that despite his error his conclusions were still good, but he had lost his authority.

Marshall Hall's next assault was equally powerful. 'Now, I come to this question of the hair,' he said. 'The position of arsenic in the hair,' he suggested, 'would not alter after death?'

William Willcox confirmed 'It would not alter after death.'

And, 'When the arsenic goes to the hair it first goes to the piece of hair nearest to the root as it grows?'

'Yes,' answered Willcox.

Marshall Hall asked the toxicologist if he had found arsenic in 'the distal end' of Miss Barrow's hair — that is, the parts furthest from her head. Yes, he conceded he had.

So, said Marshall Hall, the level of arsenic in the ends of Miss Barrow's long hair indicated that, in fact, she had had arsenic in her body over a prolonged period of time, 'And the minimum period would be something about three months?'

'I think that,' Willcox conceded.

And, Marshall Hall, continued: 'The presence of arsenic in the distal end of the hair is indicative probably of the taking of arsenic more than twelve months ago?'

'Probably,' Willcox answered.

In short, Willcox was acknowledging the likelihood of chronic arsenic in the body, since it had been there over a long period of time. Nonetheless, he continued to assert that 'one fatal dose in the last three days' had killed Miss Barrow.

At that moment, his evidence seemed remarkably like the testimony of Alfred Swaine Taylor at the trial of Dr Smethurst that had destroyed the reputation of forensic pathology fifty years earlier. Under continued pressure, he tried to cover his tracks.

'There is one point which I have not mentioned,' said Willcox, 'which rather affects these results, and that is when I took the hair for analysis [it] had been lying in the coffin, and it was more or less soaked in the juice of the body.' The arsenic, he suggested, came from the 'juice'.

Marshall Hall was scathing. He came back repeatedly in a tone of disbelief. But if there was a possibility of 'soakage' he asked, why examine the hair at all? Why not disregard it at once?

He went on to ask Willcox about the effects of arsenic if taken medicinally. 'Would that make the effect of gastro enteritis more serious to her or not?' It depended on the amount, Willcox answered, conceding that 'if it had been taken in amounts to cause irritation of the stomach, then obviously the gastro enteritis would increase'.

Marshall Hall was conducting a powerful case, and at this point of the trial he had the upper hand. But everything changed when Frederick Seddon decided, against his counsel's advice, to take the stand. As soon as he started speaking Seddon revealed himself to be an arrogant, overbearing narcissist, and his obsession with money was so extreme as to appear ludicrous. He spent nearly three days in the dock arguing in a rude and condescending manner with the prosecution lawyer, Rufus Isaacs. His attitude was particularly offensive because of Isaacs' own style, which was 'disarmingly quiet, polite and equable', and his obvious ability (the following year he was made Lord Chief Justice and in time he would become Viceroy of India). 'There was no motive for me to commit such a crime,' Seddon informed Isaacs, as though the lawyer was an idiot. 'I would have to be a greedy, inhuman monster, or be suffering from a degenerate or deranged mind, as I was in good financial circumstances.' A man with an ordered mind, plainly, would murder only when the financial incentives were more pressing.

The jury found Frederick Seddon guilty of murder, and he was sentenced to hang. There was a good deal of public unease about the verdict, and a petition was got up to secure a reprieve. More than a hundred thousand people signed it, and a public meeting in support of a reprieve was held in Hyde Park, but to no avail. Frederick Seddon was duly hanged in Pentonville prison.

As far as the forensics team was concerned, it was a thin victory. William Willcox had demonstrated some impressive science in showing the administration of so large a dose of arsenic when presented with such a tiny sample from which to work. But the Crown could not have been happy with his collapse under the pressure of a Marshall Hall broadside.

And for Bernard Spilsbury, the spectacle of Edward Marshall Hall in attack mode and William Willcox tied up in knots amounted to a useful lesson in the demands and tactics of the courtroom. He evidently thought the prosecution lucky to have won the case, and in his copy of a book on the trial of Frederick Seddon he underlined a passage in Marshall Hall's opening speech: 'the whole of the evidence in this case is totally different from the evidence in any other case of which we have any record. It is entirely constructive evidence, it is entirely argumentative evidence.' After the trial, Spilsbury said that Seddon's behaviour in the courtroom had inspired him to make a study of murderers and their vanity. Just before Seddon had been sentenced, he had appealed to the judge as a brother Mason to overturn the jury verdict. This Masonic signal, along with his constant turning towards the windows to give the press photographers a good view of his face, Spilsbury took to be signs of Seddon's arrogance and self-regard.

A year later, in April 1913, a new set of headlines appeared in the newspapers: 'Airman's Tragic Death in Flat . . . Young Woman arrested and charged with Murder . . . I shot him four times.'

Photographs of the woman, Jeannie Baxter, showed her entering Marlborough Street Court, a picture of tragic beauty. She was fashionably dressed and swathed in white furs that reached down almost as far as her little ankle-boots. Her eyes were downcast, and there was an air about her that the pressmen recorded as 'prepossessing'. A reporter inside the police court noted that Jeannie had 'a fresh complexion, and was smartly dressed in a tailor-made navy blue costume, with a large white feather boa and muff and dainty hat with an ostrich feather'. Her victim was her lover, Julian Hall, also pictured in the newspapers – a fine figure of a man, tall with broad shoulders, handsome, well-defined features and piercing dark eyes.

The case against Jeannie seemed conclusive. Around midday on 15 April several shots had been heard coming from Julian's flat in Denman Street, just off Shaftesbury Avenue. Jeannie had rushed from the flat 'crying and in a state of hysteria'. 'I have shot him,' she told Julian's neighbour Charles Caswell, 'See if you can do anything for him. He dared me to do it. Oh why did I do it, when we had arranged everything so happily for this evening?' Caswell ran next door, where a revolver and six spent cartridges were found. Julian, who was his friend, lay on the bed, bleeding from the mouth and unable to speak. Caswell held his hand until he died. He then locked Jeannie in the next door flat while he fetched a policeman.

When PC William Thornett arrived, Jeannie once more confessed: 'I did it. I shot him four times. We had arranged to do it . . .'

'I put her back in Mr Caswell's room,' said Thornett, 'and locked her in. She was in two or three minutes when I released her as I was afraid she would jump out of the window.' He next allowed her to put on a hat and furs, then took her by taxi-cab to Vine Street police station. When they arrived, Divisional Detective Albert Hawkins charged Jeannie with murder. She said, 'I am 24 and am being kept by the gentleman I shot tonight.'

A preliminary post-mortem was conducted by Dr Percy Edmunds; then on 21 April Bernard Spilsbury conducted his own autopsy. 'The body was well-nourished', he wrote, 'decomposition was just commencing. There was an open wound on the front of the chest on the right side, almost five inches vertically above the right nipple . . . Another wound was situated at the back of the chest on the left side.' He also found an entrance and exit wound on the right arm. Although Jeannie claimed to have shot Julian four times, it was clear that only two of the bullets had actually hit him. The arm wound was relatively minor, since 'the bullet had run beneath the skin without injuring either muscles or large blood vessels'. The chest wound, though, was fatal. It had passed through the lower part of the windpipe, and part of the left lung. 'It was impossible for one bullet to have caused both wounds.'

Spilsbury noted that the liver was enlarged and 'on microscopical examination showed very advanced fatty disease for which I could find no adequate cause in the body. The stomach had a slight odour of brandy and I thought it likely that the liver disease was due to excessive alcoholism.'

He then examined the pyjamas that Julian had been wearing when he died. These had been laundered after the shooting. Nonetheless, Spilsbury believed that the shape of the bullet hole, and the way the gunpowder had settled around it, provided vital evidence. For the first time in a long history of collaboration, he consulted a young gun expert, Robert Churchill. Under Churchill's supervision, he fired a gun at a piece of material 'like the pyjama jacket with pieces of leather behind to represent skin'. He did this seven times, with the gun at varying distances from the target. The first, with the muzzle of the revolver just touching the cloth, showed the fabric 'tearing, scorching and burning'. The seventh shot, at a range of three feet, produced blackening at the edge of the opening in the material, and few but widely separated powder granules.

'The leather', he wrote, 'is quite free from any change except for the hole.'

'Taking this evidence into consideration,' Spilsbury informed the police, 'and with my own experience with these experiments, and my own observations of the wound in the chest, I have formed the opinion that the revolver must have been certainly more than a foot from the chest wound when discharged, and I think it probably was about three feet and it may have been a little more . . .'

To show that the fatal wound was not self-inflicted, Spilsbury demonstrated to the police how difficult it would have been for Julian to have held the gun at the correct angle to produce the wounds that his body sustained. Holding the revolver to his own body (he and Julian were about the same height), he said: 'The hand has to be acutely flexed and loses its power and I do not think I could myself pull the trigger in this position.' More incriminating still, the distance from the revolver in Spilsbury's hand to his body was small – nowhere near the three feet away suggested by the pyjama-jacket experiments.

According to Bernard Spilsbury, Julian Hall could not have shot himself. He also asserted that the shot could not have been made 'during a struggle in which the deceased man was holding the revolver'. Percy Edmunds and Robert Churchill agreed – so the prosecution was in the fortunate position of being able to produce three expert witnesses to testify that Jeannie Baxter shot Julian Hall independently, without his help. It must have seemed an open-and-shut case, particularly to Robert Churchill, who took the view that 'no person intelligent enough to get away with murder would ever commit a murder with a firearm' because the evidence was simply too incriminating. And if someone pulled the trigger more than once it was, he thought, many times more difficult to establish an innocent motive.

The trial opened on 13 June 1913, a warm day that brought people out on to the streets of London. It was the birthday of

King George V, and the city was 'gay with flags' and packed with 'an impossible jam' of traffic, suggesting that 'a spell of sunshine breeds motor cars as it multiplies midges'. At the Old Bailey, the court was crowded with women who craned forward to see Jeannie as she entered the dock. 'They saw a slim woman', reported the *News of the World*,

> who looked scarcely more than a girl, attractively dressed in a black silk frock, cut low at the neck, with purple facings, and with white lace ruffles at the wrists and breast. A purple sash was round her waist, and round her neck a black feather boa. Her small hat of black straw was trimmed with purple flowers and a long, white feather.

While the jury was being sworn in, 'her lips began to quiver and she produced a dainty lace handkerchief to dry her tears'.

The story that unfolded was the familiar one of a woman desperate to be married. Jeannie, a young single mother (the newspapers called her a 'widow' for the sake of respectability), had met Julian in a London nightclub in August 1912. He cut a romantic figure, being handsome, wealthy and a trainee pilot who flew Bristol bi-planes over Salisbury Plain. The couple were instantly and 'violently' attracted to each other. Julian left his current girlfriend for Jeannie, and she put in jeopardy her relationship with a rich man called Mr Unwin. He, it turned out, had for the past two years been keeping Jeannie, sending her £5 a week, buying her a horse and trap, and furnishing her flat in Portsdown Road, Maida Vale, an area – less than a mile away from Bernard Spilsbury's house – known for its 'Corinthian' character, since many wealthy men kept mistresses there.

When Mr Unwin learned of Julian, he stopped Jeannie's money. Julian promised to marry her, but kept changing his mind, making her mad with worry. She had a 6-year-old daughter to support, as well as a flat to maintain and a servant to keep. Her maid, Thérèse, gave evidence at the trial, which did nothing to help Jeannie's case. According to Thérèse, Jeannie 'was visited by different men at her flat nearly every day and they spent the night there'. Julian, she said, 'used to come and spend two or three days nearly every week.' On the evening of 14 April, the night before the shooting, Jeannie had said 'that Mr Hall had spoiled everything between her and her friend Mr Unwin. Hall had promised to marry her and had to marry her now. If he wouldn't marry her, could anyone be punished very much that would shoot him dead?' Thérèse replied, 'I don't know.'

The testimony of Julian Hall's friend Charles Caswell was similarly damaging. Jeannie, he said, had asked him to get Julian (or Jack, as she called him) to marry her, or, alternatively, to get Mr Unwin to come back. 'I was at Baxter's flat about three months ago,' he said, 'when she was talking about her relations with Unwin and Hall. She was sober and serious at the time; she understood what she was saying and said it as though she meant it. She said: "Either Jack must marry me or he must get Mr Unwin back for me or I will kill Jack."' He was quite sure that on 15 April Jeannie had told him she had shot Julian and was sure she didn't say 'the thing went off'.

Edward Marshall Hall did not regard Jeannie's position as hopeless. In fact, he took on her defence with immense relish. As his biographer put it, 'he was always at his best when his case had a strong romantic interest', and he felt he had a lot to work with. Like many others, he found Jeannie a fascinating character, not least when, after interviewing her in prison, he looked out of the window into the courtyard below and saw her performing a little dance on her way back to her prison cell. He was amazed by her self-confidence. She didn't seem to think, even for a minute, that she was guilty of murder – or that anybody else would take such a dim view of her.

In court he was able to establish that Julian Hall was extremely fond of drink, had drunk a bottle and half of brandy the day before he died and was constantly talking of death. To be an airman was, in itself, a highly risky business – on the day that his death was first reported in the newspapers, there were two stories of airmen in accidents. One, Mr Gaudart, died 'when 40 feet up, the machine began to sway ominously and, after turning turtle, fell into the sea'. The other, Mr Busteed, was rescued from the Solent after his bi-plane crashed off the coast of the Isle of Wight.

Julian, it seemed, enjoyed taking death-defying risks. And, in that spirit, he kept two revolvers in a wooden chest in his flat, which he liked to take out and show off to guests. On one occasion, at Jeannie's flat, he had proposed a duel to Mr Unwin. Each man, he said, should light a cigarette. The lights should then be switched out, and they should shoot at each other in the dark using the cigarettes as a guide. Mr Unwin refused the offer. Julian then 'took the revolver and shot at Mr Unwin's photograph. The bullet went through the head of the photo and hit a bottle of champagne. Then Mr Hall shot at Mrs Baxter's photo and afterwards he pointed the revolver over his shoulder and fired backwards, through the sitting-room door.'

When Bernard Spilsbury was called to the witness stand Marshall Hall made the most of Julian's recklessness, and love of his guns. Taking the revolver, which was in the courtroom as an exhibit, he held it at arm's length and pointed it at his own chest. Might not Julian Hall have done exactly this, when Jeannie Baxter visited him on the morning of 15 April? Might he not have said 'Here, come and shoot me,' inviting a struggle for the revolver, which was fired in the ensuing confusion? Spilsbury, along with Percy Edmunds and Robert Churchill, took the firm view that he did not accept Marshall Hall's portrayal of events. The expert testimony all pointed in one direction – the fatal wound did not occur during a struggle and was not self-inflicted.

Marshall Hall now put Jeannie Baxter in the witness-box, and she gave her evidence in 'a low, clear voice'. She said that on the morning of 15 April she had arrived at Julian's flat at 8.30 in the morning and found him in bed. He kissed her good-morning, and said he had been awake since 5 o'clock, adding, 'I am fed up. I have got a fit of the blues.' She said she was sorry, and then asked about the arrangements for their marriage – she had already bought a dress. He said he hadn't done anything about the wedding, adding, 'Bill' (his name for Jeannie), 'I cannot keep my promise. It is better I should finish it. This drink is killing me, Bill, I cannot stand it.' She explained that they had had many quarrels on the subject, and that Julian had 'knocked me about.' 'Did that make you hate him?' she was asked. 'No,' she replied, 'I liked him all the more.' In fact, she added, 'I loved him better than anybody in the world.'

During the argument, she said, Julian got up and placed his revolver on the bedside table. She asked what he was going to do and he replied: 'Never you mind.' Alarmed, and believing he was about to take his own life, and perhaps hers, she pointed out that should anything happen to her, her little girl would be alone in the world. Julian then wrote out a will, leaving all his money to Jeannie for the benefit of her daughter, and the 'will' was produced in court as an exhibit. Then, said Jeannie, Julian took the revolver in his hand, 'and was whistling down the barrel'. She said she tried to take the gun from him, and in the struggle it went off, hitting him twice. Then, she said, she fired four more shots into the air to empty the chamber. When questioned, she denied having told people that she wished to shoot Julian.

The time had come for the summing-up speech for the defence. Marshall Hall, it was said, took the view that 'the strict letter of the law would rarely avail to obtain an acquittal'. Instead he preferred to appeal to the human instincts of his juries. As the journalist Theodore Felstead put it: 'As an actor, he was just superb.' And this was now the case.

Julian Hall, proclaimed Marshall Hall, had been a young man of magnificent physique, 'well dowered with this world's goods and possessed of a disregard for death which fitted him for the career of an aviator'. He had taken up a branch of national defence which would hereafter be of immense value to the country. He was a man who might have used his life to great advantage. Yet he allowed himself to be brought down by drink and passion to a level lower than some animals. The sordid facts, he said, could only be described by the pen of a Zola and the brush of a Hogarth – only they could have done justice to the life and death of a man whose tragic end had a sequel at the Old Bailey. The message was clear: Julian Hall had been the cause of his own ruination, and Jeannie had merely been caught up in the whirlwind as he crashed and destroyed himself.

The judge was persuaded by Marshall Hall's eloquence, and by Jeannie's evidence. He said he had tried to look upon the case 'from the most lenient point of view', and urged the jury to consider a verdict not of murder, but manslaughter. As the jury left the courtroom, Jeannie 'chatted vivaciously from the dock with a number of her friends, and she laughed heartily at their remarks'. After sixty-five minutes, the foreman returned. She was found guilty of manslaughter and sentenced to three years in prison. Jeannie seemed stunned, and was led weeping from the dock. But the result was, in fact, a triumph for Marshall Hall and the defence. His old-style drama, his mesmerizing presence in the courtroom, and his ability to make a fanciful version of the events seem like a convincing truth had won out over Spilsbury and the scientists.

5

Margaret

IN DECEMBER 1913 Margaret Elizabeth Lofty fell in love with a man named William Gilbert. Margaret was a 37-year-old spinster with little to recommend her on the marriage market. She was from a respectable background – her father, now dead, had been a clergyman. But she was not well off, and supplemented the family income by taking up occasional jobs as a lady's companion. For most of the time she lived in Bristol with her sister Elsie and their elderly mother. The household, it seems, was content, though not particularly happy or joyous. The sisters got along, but Margaret, according to Elsie, was 'usually depressed' and was a private, rather introverted woman. She didn't tell Elsie her secrets.

Margaret's appearance was of the buttoned-up kind. She had embraced a new fashion for women to wear a simple, sensible skirt along with a high-necked white blouse and a tie that looked as if it belonged to a man. The effect was severe and sombre and reflected the politics of the time, as women began to move into men's jobs and the militancy of the suffragettes continued to fill the newspapers. In June 1913, on the first day of Jeannie Baxter's prison sentence for the manslaughter of Julian Hall, the suffragette Emily Davison threw herself under the King's horse at Epsom, and died three days later. Margaret, as far as we know, was no suffragette, but she was a serious young woman, and the fashion for the mannish clothes of political women suited her character better than the frills, feathers and furs worn by the sexy girls who went to night-clubs and slept with handsome young aviators. It was unfortunate that the starkness of her dress was not softened by a pretty face. Instead, she had a horsey look. Her face was long, her nose and mouth were not dainty, and when she wasn't smiling she looked slightly cross, like a schoolmistress in charge of a difficult class. Besides, she looked like a working woman at a time when such a person was synonymous with being single. This all mattered, because Margaret had never given up the hope of marriage and it was a troublesome fact that potential husbands, for the most part, still preferred women who were not only young but also sweet and appealing, gentle and supremely feminine.

In 1913 *Strand Magazine* asked some well-known men their views on 'The Sort of Woman a Man Likes'. The novelist Joseph Hocking wrote:

He doesn't like a political woman and on the whole has very little sympathy for the suffragette order . . . Man's ideal of womanhood, as far as I know, is suggested by the old-fashioned word 'womanliness'. She is a sympathetic companion, one who desires to share in the joys and sorrows of her husband. She is a lover of home and children, and finds her greatest joys by the fireside.

E. Temple Thurston thought a man liked 'a woman who can minister to his selfishness without obliterating herself, who can listen to his egotism without making him feel he is monopolizing the conversation'; and F. Frankfort Moore that

She should confine herself to the language of the angels if she wishes to be liked by men . . . The women who are liked least by men are those who try to speak with the tongues of men, and the greater the success of their efforts in this direction the less they are liked by men. I plump for the woman who is kind. Men do not want a polyglot; they want one who will put the kettle on.

The illustrations that accompany the article show the 'womanly woman' as gentle and extremely pretty. The 'political woman', by contrast, points a hectoring finger, is an ugly harridan, wears a shirt and tie and has no womanly shape to her body.

Another article that year, entitled 'The Sort of Man a Woman Likes', questioned whether or not women liked their men to be tyrants. 'Whilst all women detest a bully,' thought Adelaide Arnold, 'there are many who secretly approve a master.' Marjorie Bowen agreed: 'Personally, I think women *do* like to be tyrannized over, and that the one unforgiveable thing in women's eyes is weakness of the spirit.' And Mrs Stanley Wrench's view was that 'in her secret heart woman likes to be tyrannized over, though never, even to herself will she acknowledge this. If she is in love . . . there is more of the Cave Woman in her than she imagines.' The dissenters included Sophie Cole, who wrote: 'As to being tyrannized over, I think women imagine they like it before marriage, and discover they detest it after . . . It is "understanding" which men and women have craved of each other since the time they were created so dissimilar that the aspiration is impossible of fulfilment.' Mrs H. H. Penrose was philosophical, observing that 'the average woman has never been very exacting in her demands – perhaps owing to her melancholy preponderance in the marriage market which inclines her to take what she can get and be thankful for the moment'.

When William Gilbert came along, Margaret was more than thankful – she was smitten. Their romance, much of it conducted in secret, was the most exciting event of her life so far. It later emerged that she sent him at least 220 letters. 'As far as I know this is the only love affair she ever had,' said another sister, Emily (who lived away from home and worked as a teacher). William had some income of his own but not a fortune. He had worked as a clerk for several railway companies – the Midland, the Great Eastern and then the Central, and his work had taken him to live in Sheffield, Manchester and London. He seemed to like being on the move. He was currently employed as a commercial traveller for a Sheffield-based firm; so Margaret probably saw him only now and then, when he was passing through Bristol. However, she must have thought she knew him well enough to want to marry him, because when he proposed, she accepted.

Margaret told her family of her engagement, and plans were made for a wedding at the Church of St Mary's in the Clifton area of Bristol. The Revd Norton at St Mary's wrote to the Revd Curzon, vicar of St Oswald's church in Sheffield, asking after William Gilbert. The Revd Curzon's reply contained terrible news: William Gilbert was already married. His wife was living in Sheffield but hadn't seen her husband since October – and it was now December. Margaret broke off the engagement, and wrote to Mrs Gilbert's family asking for all her letters to be destroyed. They, also distraught, complied with her request. Margaret had been utterly deceived by a cad, and had come frighteningly close to being lured into an illegal, bigamous marriage.

The following year the world changed. On 4 August 1914 Germany invaded Belgium, and that evening Britain declared war. The following day Lord Kitchener was appointed war minister, and government notices appeared in the papers, under the headline 'Your King and Country Need You', urging all unmarried men between 18 and 30 to join up and fight. By mid-August the Germans had marched into Liège, and the Kaiser had ordered the destruction of Britain's 'contemptible little army'. By the end of the month the government recruitment notices were announcing 'another 100,000 men wanted', and urged single men up to the age of 35 to enlist, along with ex-soldiers up to 45, and former officers up to 50. Soon, married men and widowers with children were also expected to do their patriotic duty. Had *Strand Magazine* now carried an article on 'The Sort of Man a Woman Likes', there would have been only one type – a soldier.

The newspapers were filled with articles about the difference between those manly men who were joining the army and the contemptible shirkers who weren't. It was no longer acceptable to be a 'nut', 'a cornerman' or a 'lounger': types who could be tolerated for their style, wit and dancing abilities in hedonistic prewar days. Now, under the headline 'cornermen', the *Daily Express* condemned the 'loafers who idle while patriots enlist', and complained about the scores of men to be seen on London streets, 'lounging about smoking pipes or cigarettes', spending all their days around the tavern doors, and scoffing at the men in khaki who were to be seen marching through the streets. The appeal to 'the manhood of the country . . . does not touch the Cornerman. Is it because he has no manhood left?' Such people were 'weak-kneed parasites'.

The *Daily Mirror* published a letter from a self-confessed 'nut' who was ready to fight. 'I am a "loafer", a "slacker", a "stroller",' he wrote. 'I actually wear a blazer, and smoke cigarettes sometimes. Also, I am at a seaside resort . . . I know for a fact that there are many like myself who are waiting to be given the chance to do their duty.' The next day, the paper declared its faith in such men:

> We are not so far inclined to join those who complain that English youth is all of the 'nut' variety, that watches football and parades the streets, news-gaping. And, besides, there is a lot to be said for the 'nut'. He wants rousing. He won't be flustered. He doesn't run round in circles when bad news comes. But once aroused, he fights well enough.

Women reluctant to offer up their husbands and sons to the battlefields of the Western Front were similarly urged to put country first. 'Every woman should be told to ask all her young men friends, "Why have you not offered yourself?",' wrote 'A. W.' in the *Daily Express*. 'Let us as mothers, sisters, sweethearts, and friends set such a cheerful example of sacrifice that no able-bodied young man may have an excuse for shirking his obvious duty under the cloak of "considering his women-folk"', wrote Beatrix Hudson Pile. According to the *Daily Mirror* it was the job of women to shame men: 'If all the girls of England refused to be seen out in the streets except with sweethearts and friends in khaki, Lord Kitchener would soon have all the men he requires.'

On 18 August a debate started after the *Mirror* carried a letter signed 'Ensign'. This began: 'As one of a certain portion of English girls who do not faint at the sight of blood, but who inherit the same martial ardour that inspires their brothers and sisters to action, I ask why can't girls go to war?' The following day, the paper wrote of 'Militancy in a New Form' – a reference to the suffragettes – and carried a letter from a lady signing herself 'medical woman', deploring the women who 'are making their sex ridiculous by learning to shoot'. This was 'making a game of a grave and grievous business'. Women in war should not take up shooting but rather be nurses: 'The power of delicate and sympathetic movements required in the nursing of the sick is more or less destroyed by strenuous exercises, such as the use of the rifle. Patients complain bitterly enough already of the rough, jerky movements of present-day nurses who have spoilt in tennis and golf their power of delicate manipulation.' A few days later, she emphasized the point. 'I have known sick children shriek at the approach of golfing or tennis-playing mothers, dreading the jar to the nerves and sensitive body which the hard, sinewy hands of these would cause.'

The image of a ministering nurse (who didn't play tennis or golf and didn't shoot) was everywhere. British hospitals sent many of their nurses off to the front, as did the suffragettes, and the *Daily Express* set up a controversial scheme for young women to do a crash course in becoming '*Express* nurses', who would, in theory at least, be of assistance to their more qualified sisters. Needlework was also part of the war effort. Women were urged to make clothes for the soldiers, and magazines carried articles on how to make bedsocks and balaclavas. The popular magazine *Home Notes* was one of several to carry a government notice headed: 'Your Country Needs You, How Women Can Help'. Women, it said, should keep calm, economize wisely, support men who enlisted and learn first aid. 'Don't Get Nervy', women were told, and 'Keep Smiling . . . A glum face helps nobody and there is no merit in looking as if all the cares of the world are on *your* shoulders. God Save the King.'

That August Margaret returned home to Elsie and her mother, after several weeks working as a 'companion'. She seemed settled back in Bristol, resuming her quiet life. Little trace remains of her activities during the following few months, other than the documents recording several visits to a solicitor and a doctor towards the end of November, in order to take out an insurance policy on her life. The doctor rated her 'a first-class life', stating on an insurance form that in general appearance she was 'thoroughly healthy'. In answer to the question 'What is the configuration of the applicant?' he replied: 'Of spare habit – well developed'. His meaning was not that she was overweight – she wasn't – but rather that she was in no way undernourished. Another question directed at Margaret was: 'What quantity and kind of stimulants do you usually take daily?' 'Am practically an abstainer', she replied. 'Or may have a glass of wine on special occasions such as Christmas Day'.

In consultation with her solicitor, Margaret insured her life for £700. The premium was £24 12s 4d. It was explained that if she were contemplating marriage, there would be an extra 35s to pay. But she said she had no plans to marry in the near future. On 11 December she called in at the solicitor's office to collect the policy. The solicitor, Mr Cooper, noticed that when she had first come to see him, she seemed quite at sea with insurance matters – but on later visits she seemed to have the business 'at her finger ends'. When they later found out about her insurance policy, her family were surprised. She hadn't told them about it.

This was odd behaviour for Margaret, but not as peculiar as her conduct on 15 December, when she left the house saying she was going out to tea but did not return. That evening, at about 7 o'clock, Elsie received an express letter, which contained two notes – one for her, and one for their mother. The letter was sent from Bristol railway station, and the first note read:

> Dear Elsie,
> I am off to a situation and meet my lady here. We go, I believe, to London for a day or two. Am looking after her while her daughter has a holiday. It is only for a short time I believe. Hope to see you soon. Will write full particulars as soon as ever I can. Don't worry, am well and happy. Sorry not to have been able to tell you before, but it was arranged so quickly and barely any time,
> Your affectionate sister,
> Peggy

The second note was similar:

> My dearest Mother,
> I have got a situation for a few days to look after a lady while her daughter is away. They are friends of Rachel's. Am well and happy. Don't worry about me. Will let you know more in a day or two. Am to meet them at Station. Shall hope to see you again soon. Love to you both,
> Peggy

It was not typical of Margaret to lie to her family – but these notes were fabrications. In reality, she was not travelling to London to meet a lady, but was setting off by train to Bath with a man named John Lloyd, intending to marry him. That day she went to the local post office and closed her account, asking to have all her money – an unimpressive £19 5s 6d – to be made available to her at a post office in Muswell Hill in north London.

Arrangements, it turned out, had been made for Margaret and John to marry in Bath, then to go on to London together as man and wife.

The movements of the mysterious John Lloyd on those few days were designed to ease matters along. He had been staying at rented rooms in Bath since 9 December, and now asked his land-lady for a second room to be available on the 15th. Then, on 14 December, he went to London to arrange rooms there from the 17th onwards. That afternoon he knocked on the door of a lodging-house at 16 Orchard Road, Highgate. The door was answered by Mrs Emma Heiss, who was staying at the property while her husband Joseph was away. They were both German subjects, and Joseph had been interned because of the war. John Lloyd had seen a card in the window, and asked whether there were any rooms available to rent. Emma Heiss remembered the encounter:

> I said, 'How many rooms do you want?' He said, 'A sitting room and a bedroom for me and my wife.' I showed him the sitting room which is on the ground floor and he asked me the price. I told him 16 or 18 shillings a week (I am not sure which). He said 'That is rather a lot, can I see the bedroom?' I showed him the bedroom and he said he liked it. As we were walking out of the bedroom he said, 'Have you a bathroom?' I said, 'Yes.' I showed him the bathroom which is on the stairs and said, 'There is no hot water but I can make you some.' He said 'It does not matter much.' He stayed and had a good look at the bath. He seemed to be measuring it with his eyes, and said to me 'This is rather a small bath, but I daresay it is large enough for someone to lie in.' He then looked at me and smiled and I said 'It is.'

Lloyd then came with Mrs Heiss into the kitchen, and agreed to take the rooms. He paid a deposit of six shillings and left, saying he would return the following Thursday with his wife. Emma

Heiss asked him for a reference, but he said: 'I have paid you six shillings and ready money is better than a reference.'

John Lloyd returned to Bristol, picked up Margaret on 14 December and arrived in Bath with her on the 15th. Their landlady recalled that, as was proper, they stayed in separate rooms but had their meals together. On 17 December Margaret married John Lloyd at the local register office. On their marriage certificate he declares himself to be a land agent, and to be 38 years of age – the same age as Margaret. The witnesses were a Mr and Mrs Fellows, who were caretakers at the register office building. That same day, the couple left Bath and went by train to London. On leaving the tube at Highgate they walked to 16 Orchard Road, where their honeymoon was to begin.

But things did not go smoothly. When Mrs Heiss, who merely lodged at Orchard Road, had told her landlady Miss Lokker that she had let the rooms, Miss Lokker had not been pleased. She did not like Mr Lloyd's failure to provide a reference, and Mrs Heiss had confessed that 'she did not like the look of the man'. 'I had previously taken in a lodger without a reference,' said Miss Lokker, 'and he had robbed me.' So when Margaret and John arrived at the property at about 3 p.m., there was an unseemly confusion. The lodgers who answered the door explained that the landlady was not in, said the room was not ready, and sent the couple away, asking them to return later, when the landlady would be back. John Lloyd was, understandably, cross – since he had travelled all the way from Bath three days earlier in order to book the room in advance. Nonetheless, he and Margaret left, returning at 5 p.m. 'He was in a temper,' Miss Lokker remembered, and angry words were exchanged, during which she asked about a reference. 'He said: "I have never heard of such a thing. I have plenty of money and a Banker, that is good enough." He said he had been everywhere abroad and had never been treated as he was being treated.' Miss Lokker had taken the precaution of summoning a policeman to the house and in the presence of

Sergeant Isaac Dennison, John Lloyd's deposit was returned to
him.

So Margaret and John now trudged the streets of Highgate in
the dark, looking for somewhere to spend their wedding night.
Before long, they found a room at 14 Bismarck Road. Louisa
Blatch was the landlady, and she showed the couple a furnished
bedroom at the back of the house on the second floor. They
asked the price, and when she offered to rent it for seven shillings
a week, they agreed to take it. 'As we were coming down from
the second floor,' said Miss Blatch, 'the woman said "Have you
a bathroom?" I said, "Yes there it is."' And she pointed out the
bathroom, which was on the first floor of the house. John Lloyd
then left to fetch the couple's luggage from the station, and Miss
Blatch asked Margaret how long they intended to stay. According
to Miss Blatch, she answered 'I do not know. I do not know
what my husband is going to do, but we are going on to
Scotland.' After John returned with the luggage, the couple went
out.

The evening of their wedding day was spent visiting Doctor
Stephen Bates, who ran a practice at 131 Archway Road,
Highgate. It was John Lloyd who spoke, saying: 'I have brought
my wife in to see you, she complains of a bad headache which
came on when we got out of the Tube station at Highgate.' Dr
Bates asked Margaret several questions, but she did not answer.
He repeated his questions, but she still didn't say anything. So,
eventually: 'I put a leading question and said, "have you really a
headache, as your husband says?" Only then did she answer:
"Yes". I asked several other questions, but still got no answer. I
then said: "have you any other symptoms of any kind?" and she
replied "No".'

The doctor thought Margaret seemed 'depressed and low-
spirited'. He also described her as 'sullen and somewhat dazed'.
When he examined her, he found that her pulse was quickened

and her temperature was 100.6 degrees Fahrenheit, which 'suggested acute illness of some kind'. He thought she might have flu, so gave her some medicine to relieve the headache and told her to let him know the next day if she were no better. The couple left, and that evening posted a letter to Margaret's family. The letter gave their address as 14 Bismarck Road, and read:

Dear Elsie and Mother,
No doubt you will be surprised to know that I was married today to a gentleman named John Lloyd. He is a thorough Christian man, who I have known since June. I met him at Bath. He was then going to Canada and returning to England in September. While he was away we kept up a correspondence and found by the tone of each other's letters that our tastes and temperaments and so forth were exactly in harmony, and as I have always been one to keep my personal affairs to myself, I said not a word to anyone about the matter . . . surely you will not blame me for doing so. It is only natural that I should do anything to secure the one I love, and I have every proof of his love for me. He has been *honourable* and kept his *word* to me in everything. He is such a nice man and I am certain that you would have liked him. That is why I regret not bringing him to see you. I hope you will forgive me for not doing so. My only fault was that I wanted to carry out my plan in my own way. After all I have only done what thousands would have done. I will tell my husband all about my relations later on and no doubt he will pay you all a visit. I am perfectly happy. I hope Mother is quite well and yourself and things are now working smoothly with the new maid. Will you be kind enough to strap my box and forward same as early as possible to the above address, as there are several articles in it I require at the present time.
With love to you both,
Yours affecty,
Peggy Lloyd

When they received Margaret's letter, Elsie and her mother were so concerned that they wrote immediately, by registered post, to Frederick Kilvington, a cousin of the Loftys, urging him to find Margaret and check that she was safe. Frederick was a solicitor, working from offices in Victoria Street, London, and when he received the letter on Saturday, 19 December, he left immediately for Bismarck Road.

The previous day – the day after her visit to the doctor – Margaret had not come down to breakfast. Louisa Blatch enquired after her when she took the breakfast to John Lloyd in the couple's rented sitting-room. He told her about his wife's ill-health and her visit to Dr Bates. Later in the morning Miss Blatch saw the couple together. 'How are you feeling, Mrs Lloyd?' she asked. But it was he who answered on her behalf, saying: 'Mrs Lloyd is better, only a little headache now.' Miss Blatch reported that 'during the morning they both went out together, and were away some time.' At about 1 p.m. they returned for dinner, bringing with them some fish for the landlady to cook. Margaret had also given her a Christmas pudding the night before – but Miss Blatch did not serve it up.

After dinner, Margaret and John again went out, and at about 3 o'clock that afternoon Margaret called in at a solicitor's office at 84 High Street, Islington. She spoke to the solicitor, Arthur Lewis, and asked if she might draw up a will. 'I asked for her particulars', said Mr Lewis, 'and she said it was very short – all to husband for him to be sole executor.' He told her he would draft the will and send it along to Bismarck Road the following day. But Margaret asked whether it would be possible to draw it up while she waited and whether she could sign it straight away. Mr Lewis told her that, yes, since it was so short, he would be able to draw it up very quickly. 'I had it typed,' he said, 'and she signed it and it was handed to her. She appeared quite calm and collected.'

That afternoon the couple returned to Bismarck Road where Louisa Blatch served them tea and bread and butter. Miss Blatch thought that Margaret seemed cheerful, and did not show any sign of depression and that she 'appeared to be quite happy with her husband'. Sometime during the afternoon, said Miss Blatch, Margaret asked if she could have a bath: 'I asked what time she wanted it. She said "about 8 o'clock".' She thought that they did not go out again that afternoon, but she did not see them again until the evening. 'At half past seven,' she said, 'I told her the bath was ready. She was then in the sitting-room with Mr Lloyd and was kneeling by the fire as if warming herself. She simply replied, thanking me. I afterwards heard her go up the stairs as if going to the bathroom on the first floor.' Miss Blatch told Margaret to take her own candle to the bathroom, since the gas in the bathroom was not used. Shortly afterwards the landlady was ironing in the kitchen when she heard someone else going up the stairs. 'A few minutes after that,' she said, 'I heard a sound from the bathroom. It was a sound of splashing. Then there was a noise as of someone putting wet hands or arms on the side of the bath, and then a sigh. The splashing and the hands on the bath occurred at the same time. The sigh was the last I heard.'

A few minutes later, however, Miss Blatch did hear something else – the mournful strains of music being played on the harmonium in the Lloyds' sitting-room. The tune she heard was 'Nearer My God to Thee', the hymn that was said to have been played on the *Titanic* as the ship went down. 'I should say the organ playing went on for ten minutes', she said. 'The next sound I heard was the front door slam.' Shortly afterwards the bell of the front door rang. Miss Blatch went to answer it and found John Lloyd on the step. According to Miss Blatch, he said, 'I forgot I had a key,' adding: 'I have been for some tomatoes for Mrs Lloyd's supper.' He then asked whether Mrs Lloyd had yet come downstairs. Miss Blatch said she had not seen Margaret, and John said he would take the tomatoes upstairs to her, and ask if she would like them.

'I heard him go upstairs', said Miss Blatch,

> and I heard him call some name. He would be perhaps half-way up the stairs when he called up. I was standing at the bottom of the stairs. He then said, 'My God there is no answer.' I do not remember what I said. He called again. I then said, 'Perhaps she has gone to her bedroom.' By this time John was at the top of the stairs, just outside the bathroom door. He called out 'there is no light . . . She is in the bath. Come and help me.'

Miss Blatch said she could not come, but she dashed up the stairs, intending to rouse a male lodger in the house, and ask him to help. She heard John call out: 'Shall I let the water off?' and she replied, 'Certainly, let it off at once.' Unable to find the gentle-man lodger, she went to the bathroom door, which was wide open. John Lloyd, she said, called out again: 'Don't leave me alone. Come and help me.' Miss Blatch went inside and found John

> in the act of getting his wife out of the bath. He was lifting her but her feet and legs were still in the bath. He said nothing. I felt her arm and found it was cold. I said 'I will fetch a Doctor and a Policeman.' He said, 'I'll go.' I said, 'No I will go myself.' He said, 'Fetch Mr Bates of Archway Road, I took her to him last night.'

Miss Blatch rushed out of the house and soon found Stanley Heath, a police constable of the Y division of the Metropolitan Police, who was on special patrol duty in Archway Road – just fifty yards away from the house. He went immediately to 14 Bismarck Road, while Miss Blatch continued down Archway Road to find Dr Bates. PC Heath arrived at about 8.15 p.m. The front door was open, and he went straight to the bathroom where he saw John Lloyd 'kneeling beside the body of a naked woman that was lying on the floor. The trunk of the body was outside the bathroom and the lower limbs inside the bathroom. He was working the arms of the woman backwards and forwards.' Stanley Heath asked whether she was dead. John Lloyd didn't answer, saying only that she had been in the bath for about an hour, adding that she had complained of pains in the head and was under the treatment of Dr Bates. The policeman covered the body with a dressing-gown that was hanging on the bathroom door, and took over from Lloyd, applying artificial respiration until Dr Bates arrived. Heath noticed that there was 'foam issuing from the mouth of the body.' He also recalled that there was about six inches of water in the bath. 'I felt it,' he said, 'and it was still warm. The plug was drawn and the water actually running away.'

When Dr Bates arrived, at about 8.20 p.m., he saw Margaret 'lying on the floor naked, except that she had a dressing-gown thrown over her, and there was a constable performing artificial respiration', while John Lloyd was standing by. Margaret was lying across the doorway, with the legs and feet just inside the bathroom. 'I examined the body,' said Dr Bates, 'and found that she was dead. The trunk of the body was cold, but not quite cold. The extremities were cold.' He thought she had been dead for at least half an hour.

Margaret's body was then carried upstairs to the Lloyds' bedroom on the second floor, where Dr Bates conducted a further examination. 'The lips,' he said, 'were blue and swollen. The whole face was congested and the eyelids swollen. When I saw the body downstairs there was froth exuding from the mouth and nostrils. I formed the opinion that death was probably due to drowning. I did not notice any external marks on the body at that time.' John Lloyd came into the bedroom, said Dr Bates, and, upon hearing that there would be an inquest, remarked: 'I hope the verdict will not be suicide, as I should not like it said that my wife was insane.'

After the doctor and the policeman had left, Louisa Blatch asked John Lloyd if he 'would like somebody to see Mrs Lloyd' – meaning a woman to lay out the body. When he answered 'no', she thought he had misheard her. After all, it was seemly to have someone in, so she asked again. But he replied: 'No, the doctor has done all that is necessary.' That night, thought Miss Blatch, John Lloyd slept in the downstairs sitting-room, while Margaret's body remained in the upstairs bedroom.

The next morning – Saturday – an undertaker, Frederick Beckett, arrived. John showed him to the bedroom on the second floor. 'The body of a woman was lying on a bed in a nude state,' Mr Beckett recalled, 'with the exception that it was wrapped in a blanket.' He remembered the conversation between the two men:

'This is my wife, and I want you to carry out funeral arrangements.'

'Are you going to purchase a grave?'

'No certainly not, I cannot afford it.'

The undertaker then offered a grave at Islington Cemetery for £4 2s 6d, but John Lloyd replied:

'Oh no, just an ordinary grave. What will that cost?'

'Ten shillings, and £7 10s the funeral.'

'That is too much.'

'Well,' said Mr Beckett, 'I'll do it for £6.10.0, that will include a glass hearse and one carriage.'

John Lloyd agreed to the terms. A little later he called in at the undertaker's office at 1 Highgate Hill, where he met Frederick Beckett's brother, Herbert. He asked Herbert to remove Margaret's body from Bismarck Road at once, as 'it is a great inconvenience to the landlady, laying there.' Herbert explained that he couldn't move the body until he had clearance from the coroner's office. This came shortly afterwards, and at about 10.30

that morning Frederick Beckett took Margaret's body to the Islington mortuary.

Later that day Margaret's cousin, Frederick Kilvington, arrived at Bismarck Road, armed with his letter from the Loftys and wanting to know about her sudden marriage. He saw the land-lady, Miss Blatch, and then John Lloyd, and learned of Margaret's death. He told John that he had come on behalf of Margaret's mother, who was very old and unable to come herself. He 'did not seem to know that she had any relatives', said Frederick, 'and pro-duced some letters . . . which purported to come from her . . . These letters seemed to say that he was her only friend.' He told John that Margaret in fact had a mother and sisters and a brother. John 'then asked whether I would like to see the body, and I said I would. I went to the mortuary and saw the body.' Afterwards, he spoke with John again, and tried to find out more about him, but could glean very little – only that he had spent time in Canada and worked as a land agent. Frederick did not learn that Margaret had taken out life insurance, or that she had made a will.

That same day, Dr Stephen Bates conducted his post-mortem. He found a small bruise on Margaret's left elbow, but otherwise no external injuries. Her skull was normal, and there was no gross haemorrhage of the brain, though many minute haemorrhages 'in the substance of the brain'. Her heart seemed normal, as did the aorta and coronary arteries. In other words, there was no evidence of a brain haemorrhage or heart attack. Her lungs were very con-gested and full of frothy foam, and the stomach contained about a pint of watery fluid and some currants. There was, he said, no sign of poison. The cause of death, in Dr Bates' opinion, was asphyxia from drowning. Although her body did not display evidence that she had fainted – he thought that 'if she had influenza that, together with a hot bath, might tend her to having a fainting attack'.

Three days later, on Tuesday, 22 December 1914, the inquest took place. Frederick Kilvington attended on behalf of the Loftys and heard the policeman, Stanley Heath, testify that there was 'no sign of a struggle or disorder' when he had arrived at the scene of Margaret's death. Dr Bates gave the results of his post-mortem, and said that he thought Margaret had died after fainting in the bath. John Lloyd told of Margaret's headache. 'She was not depressed,' he said, 'but she was not extra cheerful.' He had, he said, gone to investigate the bathroom in the presence of the landlady, Louisa Blatch.

> The door was not locked as far as I remember. There was no light in the room and I struck a match and lit the gas on the left-hand side going in. I then looked straight to the bath and saw my wife under the water. The bath was about three parts full. I don't think the water was very soiled as I could see deceased and the soap plainly.

The inquest was then adjourned until the New Year, since Louisa Blatch was disabled by a bad knee.

The coroner allowed Margaret's funeral to go ahead on 23 December. That morning John Lloyd went into Herbert Beckett's office. 'Do you wish to see the body again?' the undertaker asked. According to Mr Beckett, John Lloyd replied

> 'No, no, screw it down.' I said, 'Very well, will there be any-body else but yourself following?' He said, 'There may be another one, but if they don't turn up it does not matter, don't wait.' At this time the body was being screwed down in our private mortuary at the rear of 70 Junction Road, a few doors away . . . I sent the hearse to 70 Junction Road to fetch the body and whilst waiting for it to come along, he said, 'I don't want any walking, get it over with as quick as you can.' I said, 'Very well Sir, but we must walk a little way' – it is usual to walk at least 150 to 200 yards. The hearse came along together with one carriage. I said, 'Will you wait for your friend?' He said, 'No.' He got into the carriage alone, and we walked about 150 yards, and then went on to the Islington Cemetery, where the body was interred in a common grave.'

In fact, Frederick Kilvington turned up at the cemetery, so there were two mourners after all. After the funeral John went back to the undertaker's office to settle his bill, leaving the office with the comment: 'Thank goodness that's all over.' He then went away for a few days, telling Louisa Blatch that he was going on a cycling tour.

On 1 January 1915 the inquest into Margaret's death resumed. John Lloyd returned to Highgate and walked with Miss Blatch to the coroner's court. Frederick Kilvington also came along and, after a succinct contribution from Miss Blatch, heard the jury's verdict – accidental death due to drowning. Afterwards John returned to 14 Bismarck Road, gathered up some but not all of Margaret's belongings, and left – owing Miss Blatch ten shillings in rent.

6

Inspector Neil

DETECTIVE INSPECTOR ARTHUR Neil's flat in Archway was a ten-minute walk from Bismarck Road and five minutes from Kentish Town police station where he worked. The 1911 census shows him to be a married man. But, on the day of the census, there is no sign of a Mrs Neil at home; the only other inhabitant of the apartment being Harriet Wheeler, a 75-year-old domestic servant. Neil's published memoirs, *Forty Years of Man-Hunting*, reveal practically nothing of his personal relationships and leave the impression that the flat was just somewhere to sleep.

His reminiscences, though, are filled with enthusiasm for work, showing him to be an ambitious and conscientious police officer of the type described in *Criminal Investigation: A Practical Textbook* – a leading police manual of the time. A good investigating officer, it stated, should possess 'indefatigable zeal and application, self-denial [and] perseverance . . . nothing is more deplorable than a crawling, lazy and sleepy Investigating Officer'. The author of *Criminal Investigation* was the German expert, Hans Gross, and he cited Goethe:

> Strike not thoughtlessly a nest of wasps,
> But if you strike, strike hard.

This was Arthur Neil's style. He was dogged, determined and a master of careful preparation. Gross believed that criminal investigators should also demonstrate 'swiftness in reading men and a thorough knowledge of human nature, education and an agreeable manner, an iron constitution, and encyclopaedic knowledge'. Neil couldn't lay claim to all these qualities. Nonetheless, he was a good sort, reasonably educated and highly regarded by his contemporaries for his diligence.

In 1902 he had attracted attention by apprehending the murderer George Chapman, who was subsequently hanged for poisoning three young women. In *Forty Years of Man Hunting*, he explains that Chapman's real name was Severin Klosowski, that he had worked as a 'barber surgeon' in the medical service of the Russian army, and had lived in Whitechapel in the 1880s. Neil was convinced that Klosowski was, in fact, Jack the Ripper. 'The only living description ever given by an eye-witness of the Ripper', he states, 'tallied exactly with Chapman, even to the height, deep-sunk black eyes, sallow complexion and thick, black moustache.'

Now, thirteen years later, Neil was 47 years old and a senior officer at Kentish Town Police Station. Photographs show him to be stocky, smartly dressed, with a large, open face, intelligent eyes and a strong, firm jaw. In time, he was to become one of the 'Big Four' officers of Scotland Yard, all of them of a similar thick-set face and body type, and resembling bullfrogs. But in January 1915 he was still in the second rank, determined to move up into the first, but weighed down by the police business generated by the war. The Defence of the Realm Act of the previous year had introduced a huge number of new criminal offences. It was now against the law to discuss military matters in public or to 'cause alarm'. Restricted pub opening hours were to be policed, as were curfews; and people were forbidden to buy binoculars, light bonfires, ring church bells, use invisible ink when writing abroad, and much else. Women suspected of having a sexually transmitted disease could be stopped by the police and compulsorily referred for a gynaecological examination. In addition, the *Police Gazette* was carrying lists of 'deserters and absentees from His Majesty's Service' who needed to be found; and there was much work to be done rounding up Germans for internment. In 1914 the police had been told to suspend all their annual leave and were now working six days a week on low pay.

In January 1915 Arthur Neil was 'up to my eyes in work' produced by the war. 'I was in the thick of interning aliens and other exhaustive and complicated enquiries,' he wrote. Then, one evening, 'I was turning over the various papers one by one, when my attention was attracted to an official memorandum, on which were the words – Suspicious Deaths.' Attached to the memo were two press cuttings. The first was from the *News of the World*, and read: 'FOUND DEAD IN BATH, Bride's Tragic Fate on Day after Wedding'. It related the 'particularly sad cir-cumstances' under which Margaret Lloyd met her death, and reported Dr Bates' opinion that she died accidentally in the bath. A bout of influenza, together with a hot bath, it said, 'might have caused an attack of syncope'.

The second cutting was headlined 'BRIDE'S SUDDEN DEATH IN BATH. Drowned after Seizure in a Hot Bath', and related the circumstances of Alice's death a year earlier in a Blackpool boarding-house. Dr Billing's post-mortem results were reported. Alice Smith had died accidentally as a result of her heart being 'enlarged and affected'. The doctor, according to the newspaper, 'concluded that the heat of the water had acted on the heart and caused either a fit or a faint, and in her helplessness she was drowned'.

Alice's father had seen both reports, been struck by the similar-ity of the deaths, and had contacted the Aylesbury police, who then turned to Scotland Yard. The letter from Aylesbury police had been forwarded to Inspector Neil, since Bismarck Road was on his patch. Charles Burnham, it stated, 'entertains the opinion that foul play had taken place, but as a post mortem was held he thought it useless to have further enquiries made . . . Mr Burnham has very little knowledge of the man Smith, but he describes him as about 5 feet 10 inches in height, brown eyes, walks with knees slightly bent together and feet out.'

Arthur Neil put the documents into his basket, intending to deal with the matter himself rather than pass it to a junior. The following day was entirely occupied with war business, but in the evening he took up the memorandum, and started his enquiries. He visited the police station at Upper Holloway and looked through the 'The Occurrence Book' to find the report of the uniformed constable who had been called to the scene of the death of Margaret Lloyd. 'I immediately sent for him off his beat', wrote Neil, 'and had a talk with the officer about the thing.'

PC Stanley Heath told Neil of his concern when, on arriving at 14 Bismarck Road, he had found the woman 'absolutely nude, lying on the floor'. 'I turned to the husband', said Heath, 'and said – "In pity's name, get something and cover the poor creature – don't leave her lying like this." ' Arthur Neil was left with a bad impression of the impropriety of the situation and of the unseemly behaviour of a bereaved husband, who had shown no concern for his wife's modesty.

He decided to visit the house in Bismarck Road, where he 'at once got busy' examining the bath in which Margaret had died: 'If anyone can get drowned in a bath like this, I thought, it's a marvel. The more I studied it, the more I was convinced it was a physical impossibility.' He went looking for Dr Bates but he was out on his rounds, so Neil tracked down the undertaker, Mr Beckett, who 'confidentially informed me that Lloyd appeared to be utterly callous at the funeral'. The husband, said Mr Beckett, had insisted on the cheapest coffin available, a plain elm casket, and had haggled over the price of the brass fixtures.

Very soon afterwards, Arthur Neil received another memorandum from Scotland Yard. A second man, Joseph Crossley of Blackpool, had read about the same two deaths in the newspapers, been struck by the coincidence, and had contacted his local police station. Chief Constable Pringle of Blackpool then alerted Scotland Yard. The husband of Alice Smith, who died in Blackpool, wrote Pringle, had described himself as a man of independent means, and yet he 'obtained several copies of the death certificate from the Registrar, which would make it appear that he had her insured in several insurance companies'. Pringle also thought it suspicious that Mr Smith had had his wife buried in a common grave, and in a plain deal coffin. He urged Scotland Yard to find out whether George Smith and John Lloyd were the same man.

In the next few days Arthur Neil interviewed the Highgate landlady, Louisa Blatch, the doctor, Stephen Bates and Margaret Lloyd's cousin, Frederick Kilvington. Miss Blatch, he said, had thought the behaviour of the Lloyds 'very normal'. She had no idea that they were so recently married. As for the circumstances of the death, there had been 'very little time' in which Lloyd might have played a role in his wife's death. She had heard him playing the organ and going out to buy tomatoes, and had been with him when, back from his shopping trip, he discovered his wife dead in the bath. There was no sign of a struggle. Mr Kilvington had thought the coroner conducted 'a very careful enquiry into the case, and he failed to see how the jury could return a different verdict to the one they did'. However, Arthur Neil noted that, at the inquest, very few questions were put by either of the solicitors present and that the coroner was in favour of an open verdict, partly because of the lack of evidence as to what had happened, and partly because 'so little was known about the parties'.

In his police report of 19 January, Neil writes that Police Sergeant Isaac Dennison, who had happened to see John Lloyd, described him as 'a man about 40, height 5 feet 9 and a half, complexion and build, medium, full dark moustache'. This description, says Neil, somewhat agrees with the description of the man Smith, supplied by Mr Burnham . . . but [neither] the Police Sergeant nor any of the persons who saw Lloyd are able to say whether there was any peculiarity about his legs or feet, as described by Mr Burnham of the man Smith, although PC Stanley Heath . . . does think there was a peculiarity about his legs.

The case, concluded Neil, 'is not without an element of suspicion, having regard to the similarity of the two cases, though both may have been accidental deaths and simply a remarkable coincidence'.

Nonetheless, he decided to find out whether John Lloyd and George Smith were the same man – not an easy task. There were no known addresses for or photographs of John Lloyd, and Frederick Kilvington was very anxious that no enquiries be made of Margaret's mother and sister at Bristol, 'as they are greatly distressed'. The best way forward, thought Neil, was to obtain tracings of the signatures of Lloyd and Smith from the marriage registers – though at this point he did not know where George Smith and Alice Burnham had been married. He suggested also that further descriptions be obtained from Charles Burnham in Aston Clinton and Joseph Crossley in Blackpool.

Arthur Neil soon learned that Margaret Lloyd had taken out a life insurance policy with the Yorkshire Insurance Company of Bristol. This information led him to Thomas Cooper, the joint manager of the insurance office. Inspector Tanner of the Bristol police called on Mr Cooper, who confirmed that Margaret had taken out the policy after a visit on 24 November 1914. Mr Cooper had received notification from his London office that Margaret had died and had been informed that probate of her will had been obtained by Mr W. P. Davies, a London solicitor, who had asked for a payment of £700 for his client, John Lloyd. Margaret, said Mr Cooper, had told two lies on her form – she had claimed that she had no intention of getting married, and had also declared herself to be of independent means. In fact, her death revealed that she was dreadfully poor. Apart from the £700 insurance money, she had left an estate of only £5.

Thanks to Mr Cooper, Arthur Neil now had a direct line of contact to John Lloyd through his solicitor Walter Davies. But he was worried that Davies might tell Lloyd that the police wished to find him. Then, if Lloyd and Smith were, indeed, the same person, he might simply change his name again and disappear.

Inspector Neil asked Mr Cooper to delay the payment of the insurance money. 'Although we have no real grounds for suspicion that the death was otherwise than accidental', Neil reported, 'something has come to our knowledge which makes it desirable to institute further enquiry as to the antecedents of Lloyd, respecting whom nothing is known, and it is desirable that he should not have the money in question for a while.' Having few other options, he then took the risk of contacting Walter Davies, who had an office at 60 Uxbridge Road in Shepherd's Bush. On 22 January, Neil reported that the solicitor 'is, confidentially, assisting us as far as is compatible with his legal position'.

Davies gave the police an address in west London for his client, but this was found to be a temporary residence, and there was no sign of Lloyd. Maddeningly, Lloyd had visited his solicitor's office within the past few days and had been annoyed that his money was not ready, and then had vanished. Davies had told him that further documents were required. It could not be long, thought Neil, before Lloyd returned.

Arthur Neil's contact with Alice's father, Charles Burnham, proved fruitful. He found out that, from the moment they were married, George Smith had tried to get his hands on Alice's money. Mr Burnham had kept George Smith's aggressive letters and now passed them over to the police. Though Smith 'was married to Miss Burnham some weeks before her death', wrote Inspector Neil, 'it is significant that she died shortly after the money – £100 – had been forwarded'. In addition, he reported,

'Mr Burnham understands that his daughter's life was insured after marriage.'

Neil was now convinced that George Smith and John Lloyd were the same man – and that, at the very least, he had acted most suspiciously. 'Well into the night I pondered and turned the thing over in my mind', he wrote. 'Yes! Tomorrow I would see the Assistant Commissioner and explain. Which was done. And a few days afterwards I was summoned to see the Director of Public Prosecutions.' The DPP, Sir Charles Mathews, did not share the detective's conviction. Arthur Neil remembered him saying, 'the idea's preposterous. A verdict of accidental death returned at Blackpool, and the same thing in London. Why, in the face of it, the thing – legally – is impossible.' However, he told Neil to carry on with his investigations.

So Inspector Neil organized a stake-out of Walter Davies' office on the Uxbridge Road, with the idea of apprehending John Lloyd when he turned up to find out about his money. The team of officers Neil selected for the task included Detective Inspector George Cole, Sergeants Frank Page and Harold Reed and Police Constable Stanley Heath. The idea was to conduct all-day surveillance – a task that was made unpleasant by the bitterly cold weather. The operation 'necessitated the strictest secrecy and intelligence to prevent the suspect from gaining the slightest intimation that any enquiry was being made'. It was a great help when Frederick Saltmarsh, who managed The Telegraph pub on the other side of the road from Davies' office, recognized Arthur Neil in the street, asked him what he was up to, and said, 'Well if I can be of any assistance, please do not be afraid to ask me.' Neil took advantage of Mr Saltmarsh's offer and made use of the first-floor room over the pub, which offered a direct view of the solicitor's premises. Only one officer now needed to be out in the cold at any time, and as a result, 'suspicion was not created in the minds of people in the vicinity and their curiosity was not aroused'.

At the same time Neil arranged for Charles Burnham to come

from Aston Clinton, in the hope that he would be able to iden-
tify Lloyd as the man who had married Alice. Mr Burnham duly
arrived, accompanied by his son-in-law. On 24 January Arthur
Neil wrote: 'I have closely questioned Mr Burnham and his son-
in-law with regard to the general appearance, habits etc. of
"Smith" and there is not a shadow of doubt but he is identical
with "Lloyd".' In fact, he was so sure of his case that he went to
see the Director of Public Prosecutions again – this time with a
view to obtaining an order for the exhumation of the body of
Margaret Lofty. However, he wrote in his police report: 'I would
respectfully suggest that it be held over pending the arrest of
Lloyd, as if it becomes public, through a new inquest being held,
Lloyd would abscond.'

The stake-out began, with Neil still on tenterhooks, worrying
that John Lloyd would notice the police presence and disappear. As
the days went by the Kentish Town police got together the documents they would need to hold Lloyd on a charge of forgery,
relating to the false name that Neil believed was on at least one of
his marriage documents. The days passed, though, with no sign of
Lloyd, and Neil decided to tell Charles Burnham and his son-in-
law to return to Buckinghamshire. Apart from the impracticability
of keeping Mr Burnham in Shepherd's Bush indefinitely, he was
concerned that Lloyd would spot and recognize Burnham first,
before the police spotted *him*.

On Monday, 1 February 1915, police officers Arthur Neil and
Sergeant Harold Reed were in the room over the pub. Sergeant
Frank Page and a local constable were out in the street when, just
after midday a man matching the description of John Lloyd
walked along the busy road, stopped at no. 60, and went into
the building. 'Page', wrote Neil, 'gave me the long-looked-for
signal, a conveying to the nose of both watchers of their pocket
handkerchiefs. I now got down hurriedly to the scene of the
active "kick-off". "You stand by me Page"', I said to my sergeant,
'and you others be ready to act, in case he has a gun on him.'

They waited for about half an hour and watched as he came out again. Harold Reed's police report states that they approached the man.

Reed asked, 'Are you Mr Lloyd?'

'Yes', he answered, 'that's me.'

Arthur Neil then came up and asked the same question, 'Are you John Lloyd?'

He answered, 'yes'.

Neil said: 'Your wife died in a bath at Bismarck Road Upper Holloway, on the 18 December last – the day after she was married to you.'

He said, 'Quite right'.

Inspector Neil then said, 'You are also said to be identical with George Smith, whose wife died under similar circumstances on December 13th at Blackpool and to whom you were only married a few weeks.'

He replied: 'Smith. I'm not Smith, I don't know what you are talking about.'

In early 1915, as the quiet drama of the Shepherd's Bush police operation was unfolding, the rest of Britain had other matters on its mind. On 19 January Zeppelin airships attacked East Anglia. 'Two persons killed and some injured at Yarmouth, Attack on the King's home at Sandringham, Bombs dropped on Cromer and Sheringham, Baby victim at Kings Lynn. The long-expected Zeppelin raid on English shores has occurred.' Zeppelin attacks had been anticipated since the war began, and much feared. Britain had no equivalent of the German giants of the sky, and nobody knew how much damage they would inflict. They might, many thought, herald the first serious invasion of Britain since 1066. They might be the harbingers of a new level of terror in an already terrible war – transporting the horror from the killing fields of France to the mainland of Britain.

The Zeppelins were a powerful symbol of German technological power. They were awe-inspiring, lighter-than-air vessels that could lift several tons and carry a crew of eighteen people along with the bombs that could be thrown overboard. They could fly higher than the flimsy heavier-than-air British aircraft that were barely strong enough to carry the pilot and one passenger. In December 1914 the *Daily Express* caught the public mood of fear by publishing on the front page a mocked-up picture showing a Zeppelin hovering over the Houses of Parliament. A few days later the *Daily Mirror* presented the airships as unassailable rulers of the sky. The British aeroplane pilots who attempted to bring them down were pictured as being as useless as 'flies against a window-pane'.

Admiral Sir Percy Scott, who was in charge of defending London against the Zeppelins, later acknowledged that he was in fact powerless against them. 'There were no guns which could fire to the height of a Zeppelin', he wrote, 'and the ammunition supplied to the guns was quite unsuitable, and was more dangerous to the people in London than to the Zeppelins above.' Also, there were no available airmen who could fly at night, 'and even if [we] had had them they would have been of no use, as there was no ammunition suitable for attacking Zeppelins'.

On 12 December the *Daily Express* reported that an English lady, Miss Kirby, who had just returned from Germany, had 'heard highly placed officials talking of a Zeppelin raid on England with a hundred airships, capable of firing projectiles from the sides, top or bottom'. And, the newspaper told its readers, Count Zeppelin had 'promised the Kaiser to make an aerial raid on England, and especially on London before the end of the year'. Rumours were rife. The novelist Marie Belloc Lowndes wrote to her mother saying, 'I do *not* believe in either Zeppelins or an invasion.' But, she said, the well-known war correspondent Colonel Repington *did* believe in an invasion of 200,000 men landing at different places.

On 16 December 1914 the seaside towns of Scarborough, West Hartlepool and Whitby had been attacked from ships at sea. Like the other papers, the *Daily Mirror* devoted its front page, and all the following pages, to the news: 'Great Britain Bombarded . . . The Germans have kept their word and carried the war to Britain's shores.' When the Zeppelins came in January, the damage done was far less than that of the earlier attack from the sea – but the imagery of Zeppelins over England was more sinister. Never before had invaders been able to occupy British sky, casting shadows over British streets, and dropping bombs on British towns. They appeared like great floating monsters, 500 feet long and forty-five feet wide, dropped their bombs, then retreated across the North Sea to their bases in northern Germany. It was a new type of warfare.

The inhabitants of Yarmouth watched as the air-ship passed close to the Britannia Pier and over Norfolk Square garden, where a bomb was dropped, before it headed off towards St Peter's Road and dropped more bombs. An eye-witness said the airship 'flew so low that he felt almost as if he could hit it by throwing stones'. Others reported (wrongly) that the Zeppelins had been guided on their route by motor cars on the ground. Spies, it was said, were at work. In Germany the news of the raid was greeted in triumphalist tones. 'Now the first Zeppelin has appeared in England', reported the *Kölnische Zeitung*,

> and has extended its fiery greetings to our enemy. It had come to pass, that which the English have long-feared and repeatedly have contemplated with terror. The most modern air weapon, a triumph of German inventiveness and the sole possession of the German Army, has shown itself capable of crossing the sea and carrying the war to the soil of old England!

It was only a matter of time, people thought, before the Zeppelins attacked London.

★

When war broke out, Bernard Spilsbury offered his services to the armed forces. The War Office, though, told him to stay in London – possibly because he had never worked as a doctor treating living people, and his expertise in forensics was hardly a priority at the Front. So he continued at St Mary's. Because of the Zeppelin threat he dispatched his wife and two small children to the Worcestershire countryside, while he devoted himself, more intensely than ever, to his work. It was his habit, on returning home to St John's Wood, to eat a quick meal before climbing the stairs to the laboratory at the top of the house. Here he would carry on working, examining the specimens that he had brought with him from mortuaries or the post-mortem room at St Mary's.

That January, Spilsbury's colleague William Willcox received a visit from Detective Inspector Arthur Neil, who explained that he believed the recent death of Margaret Lofty was suspicious, and that he wished to exhume her body. The Home Office, he said, had authorized the exhumation and had requested that William Willcox undertake an analysis of the viscera (the main abdominal and chest organs). Willcox told Neil that he need not worry about the exhumation taking place immediately. A delay of a few days or a week would make no difference. Willcox, though, was due to go to France later that year, so it was decided that Spilsbury should be the lead pathologist in the case.

When John Lloyd told Arthur Neil that he was not the same person as George Smith, the Inspector informed him that he would be detained pending identification by Alice's father, Charles Burnham. 'In that case', he replied, 'I may as well say my proper name is Smith, and my wife died at Blackpool. The entry in the [marriage] register at Bath is not correct, but that is all you can put against me.' The two deaths, he told the police, were 'a phenomenal coincidence'. Police Sergeant Harold Reed took Lloyd to Kentish Town Police Station in a taxi-cab. On the way, said Reed, Lloyd said: 'You may think it strange, but it was the irony of fate that my two wives should have died in the same way. I suppose this has come about through the insurance, but I did not know she was insured until after she was dead, or that she had made a will. Someone at Bristol – no Bath – sent the papers to me at Highgate and that was the first time I knew about the insurance. I suppose this trouble would have come when my first wife died if she had been insured.'

Within twenty-four hours of Lloyd being detained, the police found out that his real name was the one he had used in marrying Alice – George Joseph Smith – and that he was born on 11 January 1872 at 90 Roman Road, Old Ford, Bethnal Green. They also ascertained that Alice's life had, indeed, been insured for £500. 'After the marriage', wrote Inspector George Cole, 'she made a will in favour of her husband, the prisoner, and he succeeded in obtaining the full amount from the insurance company.' The police enquiries also revealed that less than a month before Alice had taken out the policy, George Smith had bought an annuity from the same company – the purchase price being £1,300. 'It is very important that we should now obtain the full particulars as to where the £1,300 came to Lloyd's Bank from', wrote Cole, 'as it is thought that it is the result of other dealings with insurance companies.' The inspector put a constable on the job of finding out all he could about Smith's financial transactions. Arthur Neil wrote: 'To my mind, this man has no regular employment and I am of the opinion that he has been obtaining his living by victimising women.'

On 2 February 1915, George Smith was charged with 'causing a forged entry to be inserted in the Marriage Register at Bath, by describing himself as John Lloyd when he was married to Margaret Elizabeth Lofty'. George's response was to say that he was guilty of no other charge. He was sticking to his declaration that the similarity of the two deaths was a remarkable coincidence; and said that Margaret had known of the circumstances of

Alice's death and had suggested that he change his name with a view to 'making a fresh start'.

The following day the front page of the *Daily Express* carried an exclusive story: 'Dramatic Arrest of Husband in London, False Entries'. The rest of the paper was filled with stories of Zeppelins, the Front and the regular appeal for new recruits to the army:

> Who has made this little island the greatest and most powerful Empire the world has ever seen. *Our forefathers*. Who ruled this Empire with such wisdom and sympathy that every part of it — whatever race or origin — has rallied to it in its hour of need? *Our fathers*. WHO will remember us with pride and exultation and thankfulness if we do our duty today? *Our children*. Justify the faith of your fathers and earn the gratitude of your children. *Enlist today!* God Save the King.

To enlist was to be a true man — patriotic and courageous.

The following day's paper carried similar messages alongside the contrasting story of a man who was a disgrace to his sex — George Joseph Smith. The front-page headlines were: 'NEW OUTRAGE BY THE HUNS' (as a submarine attacked a hospital ship), 'BREAD RIOTS' (predicted in Germany) and 'TWO BRIDES FOUND DEAD IN BATHS'. The *Express*'s reporter described George as he stood in the dock at the police court charged with making a false entry in the marriage register:

> He is a well-set up, slim, alert-looking man of medium height, with rather small, quick eyes, a prominent thin nose, dark hair brushed across his forehead, and a full, drooping, sandy moustache. His cheeks are rather hollow, and his cheek-bones stand out. Smith had little colour in his face yesterday. He listened very keenly to the evidence, with his head thrown back in an attitude of strained attention.

It was clear to all that the police were thinking of bringing a murder charge against this man.

Arthur Neil's problem was the slippery nature of the evidence.

Each of the two inquests had concluded that death was accidental. Each had occurred in a house in which other people were present, nobody had heard or seen anything untoward, and the police officers who came to the scene had observed no signs of a struggle. It didn't add up. How was it possible to drown someone with nobody noticing?

Inspector Neil threw himself into the case with 'indefatigable zeal', his first action being to accompany Bernard Spilsbury to the exhumation of the body of Margaret Lofty. He records that

the examination took place in a quiet little spot in Summer's Lane, Friern Barnet, the body being brought there by hearse, after we had seen it up from its grave. This was done in order to escape publicity, as everyone thought Spilsbury would make his examination at the local mortuary in Islington. After the test had been made by the great pathologist, Sergeant Reed and I took the coffin back to the cemetery near Finchley, paying our respect to the dead with bared heads as the sextons lowered the earthly remains of Margaret Elizabeth Lofty to her resting-place.

Despite Neil's attempt to keep the exhumation secret, it was reported in full in the *Daily Express* the following day:

BRIDE'S BODY EXHUMED, SECRET CEREMONY IN LONDON CEMETERY, MIDNIGHT SCENE.

The body of Margaret Elizabeth Lloyd who was found drowned in a bath at Highgate on the evening of the day following her marriage, was exhumed at midnight on Wednesday in East Finchley cemetery.

The exhumation was carried out with great secrecy. Only a few officials were present. They included Dr Spilsbury, the Home Office analytical expert, Divisional Detective Inspector Neil, and two other detectives, and certain witnesses who were there to establish the identity of the body after its removal from the grave to the mortuary.

The grave was a plain one, with no tombstone yet in position. The operations of the gravediggers, who worked by the dim light of lanterns, were completed at 11.30 p.m.

Shortly before midnight the coffin was brought to the surface. After the police, by a glance at the plate, had satisfied themselves that it was Mrs Lloyd's coffin, it was again lowered just below the mouth of the grave where it was allowed to rest on a temporary staging.

MORNING REMOVAL

The grave was then covered with boards and was guarded throughout the night. At half past seven yesterday morning the coffin was taken away.

Certain organs of the body were afterwards placed in receptacles and sealed and then removed for examination by Dr Spilsbury . . .

Bernard Spilsbury's case-card for the Margaret Lofty postmortem states that the body was clothed in a white flannelette nightdress, and despite a putrefactive smell, its condition was good. He found three small recent bruises on the back of the left arm which, he thought, had been caused within twenty-four hours of death. Apart from these, there were no outward signs of violence. His internal examination found that the less decomposed parts of the brain were 'congested', there was nothing to be said about the state of the lungs or air passages, since they had been opened at Dr Bates' post-mortem, and were now 'shrunken'. The tongue, he noted, was not bitten. His observation that the hymen was 'lacerated each side' suggests that Margaret had been a virgin when she had married John Lloyd, but that she had sex on her wedding night. There was no sign of poisoning.

On 8 February Inspector Neil went to Blackpool for the exhumation of Alice's body. The press, he acknowledged, 'had got full wind of my business in Blackpool, and I could see that my movements were shadowed everywhere'. In fact, he saw two or three well-known London crime reporters at various spots on his way from the local police headquarters to meet Bernard Spilsbury at Blackpool railway station. 'I admire the English Press reporter, if for nothing else but his tenacity of purpose', wrote Neil.

> Many of them, to my way of thinking, are, in experience as good as the next best Yard man any time, in regard to getting down to rock-bottom facts. In many ways they are like police detectives, they may know more than they are permitted to tell, but nevertheless, they know. In this case all of them had me set. For although the exhumation took place at the Blackpool Cemetery at the dead of night, they knew, as the contents of their papers the next morning revealed.

Bernard Spilsbury's case-notes for the Blackpool exhumation make it clear that his task was grim and of limited use. 'Coffin plain pitch pine', he writes. 'Lid sunken and crack along it. Coffin three quarters full of dirty foul smelling water with fragments of tissue which had separated from legs and feet. Clothed in white nightdress. Rotten.' The body was in a very advanced state of decomposition, the head 'almost separated from the trunk', the eyes and nose gone, and some tissues completely separated from the bones. Subcutaneous fat everywhere was 'completely converted into adipocene'. It was hard to tell from this foul mush whether heart trouble had, as Dr Billings thought, contributed to Alice's death. There was little left of the heart muscles. However, Spilsbury recorded that the body was 'very stout', that a mitral valve was 'slightly thickened', and left and right heart valves were 'extremely fatty'. Despite these observations, he wrote: 'No heart disease adequate to account for syncopal attack.' He found no evidence of poisoning, and acknowledged that it was 'impossible to give cause of death'.

The case-card suggests, though, that Spilsbury felt he might have something to contribute on other aspects of Alice's final moments. He has written down the dimensions of the bath in which she died – it was only three foot nine inches in length at its base, and one foot two inches wide at the base of the broad end, and one foot at the base of the narrow end. He has also written down the measurements of Alice's body, in particular her buttocks – indicating that she would have had difficulty fitting into the bath at all, let alone drowning in it. Further notes reflect Dr Billing's memory of arriving at the scene of Alice's death. Spilsbury has written, 'Floor much splashed with water . . . made a great spread. Smith out of breath when he brought eggs for breakfast.'

Somewhere along the way, the Dr Billing's version of events had become more dramatic and suspicious than that which he gave at the inquest. However, it still fell short of being the 'signs of a struggle' that would be clear evidence of murder.

7

The Others

TWO DAYS AFTER the exhumation at Highgate, Superintendent Heard of the Kent constabulary sent a note to the Commissioner of Police at New Scotland Yard. On 13 July 1912, he wrote, the wife of a man named Henry Williams was found dead in a bath at 80 High Street, Herne Bay. The woman's maiden name was Bessie Mundy. An inquest had been held, and jury had returned a verdict of death from misadventure. As this case appeared similar to the two cases with which John Lloyd was connected, Heard continued, 'I should be glad if you would forward me a photo and description of "Lloyd" so that I may make enquiries.' The news of Bessie's death reached Inspector Neil on 8 February 1915, as he arrived in Blackpool.

There was an outside chance that two similar deaths had been an amazing coincidence – but three was inconceivable. It was vital to establish as soon as possible that Henry Williams was the same person as George Smith, and by 10 February Inspector Neil's team had received a photograph of 'Williams'. Unlike Smith, he was clean-shaven – and though there was a resemblance to the man in police custody, it was impossible to be sure it was him. Inspector Neil sent a photograph of Smith to Herne Bay, where Williams' solicitor said he thought it was the same man, but would not swear to it. On 15 February the solicitor, along with Mr and Mrs Millgate, the next-door neighbours of Bessie and Henry, came to London. That day they identified Arthur Neil's prisoner as Henry Williams.

Under the Inspector's direction, the Kent police set about investigating the other circumstances of Bessie's death, to see how closely they matched the last days of Alice and Margaret. It soon emerged that five days before she died Bessie had made a will in favour of her husband, by which he had inherited £2,579 13s 7d. Otherwise, there was nothing to suggest foul play. The local doctor, Frank French, had testified that he had treated Bessie for epilepsy, and had said he thought that she had died from drowning following an epileptic fit. When asked 'Did you see any signs of a struggle?' he had replied 'None.' A jury had thought the death accidental and the Herne Bay coroner, Rutley Mowll, had not even thought it necessary to ask for a post-mortem. In English law a man could be brought to trial only for a single murder at a time and this, like the others, was utterly devoid of satisfactory incriminating evidence. In the circumstances, Inspector Neil thought it wise, once again, to ask the Home Office for permission to exhume a body.

The news of Bessie's death in a bath broke in the national press, and a photograph of Bessie and Henry on their wedding day was widely published. The reports caused a general stir, but were particularly shocking for a 43-year-old domestic servant named Alice Reavil, who thought that she knew the man in the photograph as Charles Oliver James. On her own initiative, she went along to look at him at Bow Street police court. Her suspicions were confirmed, and she contacted Inspector Neil.

Five months earlier Alice had left her home in Plumstead, south-east London, for a holiday in Bournemouth on the south coast. She said:

> On 7 or 8 September I was in the gardens on the front, sitting on a seat, when a man came and spoke to me. He said 'Good morning' and passed some remark about the weather . . . We had some conversation, in which he said he admired my figure. After about an hour's conversation, in which he informed me

he was an artist and had £2 a week from some land in Canada, he made an appointment for 6 p.m. the same evening. I met him, as arranged, on the pier-front.

After that, she met 'Charles' every evening for the rest of her holiday.

> After the third or fourth day of our acquaintance, he asked me to marry him. I consented, and he said he would put his money with mine and he would open an antique shop somewhere in London, probably Crystal Palace way. He asked me how much money I had, and I said I had £70 odd and some furniture, including a piano. He asked me to sell them and I decided to.

On 17 September 1914 they were married at the register office in Woolwich, near Plumstead – this was nine months after the death of Alice Burnham, and three months before the death of Margaret Lofty. Charles and Alice moved into rented rooms in Battersea Rise. Soon after, he asked her to withdraw all her money from the bank and give it to him for safe-keeping. 'On 22 September,' said Alice, 'we left the house . . . We got on a tram-car and on the way he spoke of Halifax, Nova Scotia, and asked me if I would like to go.' The newly-weds left the tram at Brockwell Park in Herne Hill and strolled through the gardens. After a while, Charles asked Alice to wait for him while he went to the lavatory. She stayed in the park for about an hour but he did not return, so Alice went back to the rented rooms where she found a telegram addressed to her, stating simply 'Wait home for letter next post'. A few hours later, a letter arrived:

> Dearest,
> I could not possibly let you before hand know my program otherwise you may not have agreed to have come together untill my return from Halifax. But I am due to be at Halifax Canada next Friday – also I could not bear to come and say good bye before going because you woud perhaps have broken down and tried to stop me from going so I thought it best to do

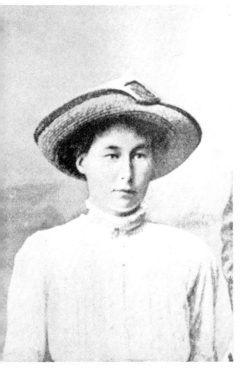

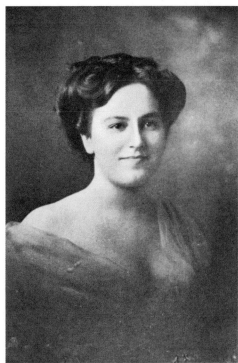

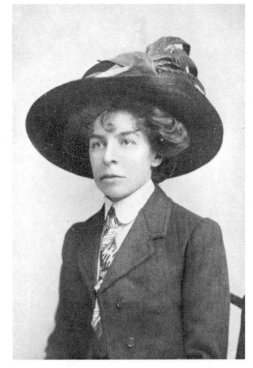

Above left: Bessie Mundy, who married Henry Williams in Weymouth in 1910. She was 'easily led', said her brother, Howard

Above right: Alice Burnham, the spirited young woman who in 1913 left a nursing career to marry a man of 'independent means'

Right: Margaret Lofty. In December 1914 she secretly married John Lloyd. The couple spent their wedding night in a Highgate lodging house, with a bath

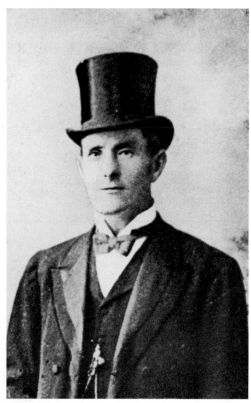

Left: Henry Williams looking dashing on the day of his marriage to Bessie Mundy

Below: George Joseph Smith. 'When he looked at you for a minute or two you had the feeling that you were being magnetised'

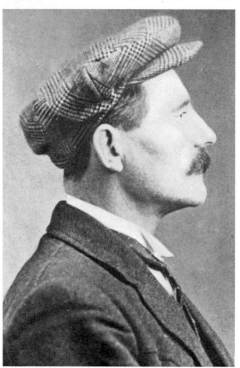

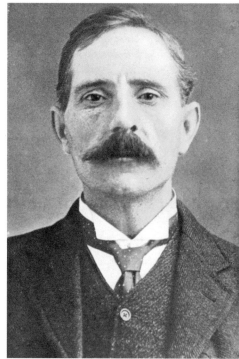

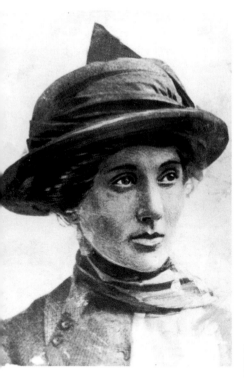

Left: Alice Reavil, a domestic servant. She met Charles Oliver James during her holiday in Bournemouth and married him in September 1914

Right: Edith Pegler, who answered George Smith's advertisement for a housekeeper in 1908. He told her that he had money and wished to settle down, and asked her to marry him

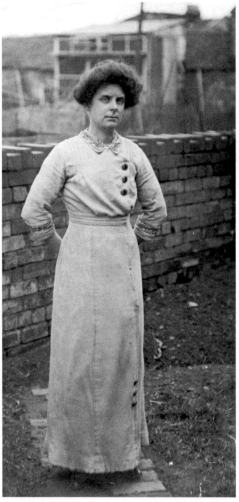

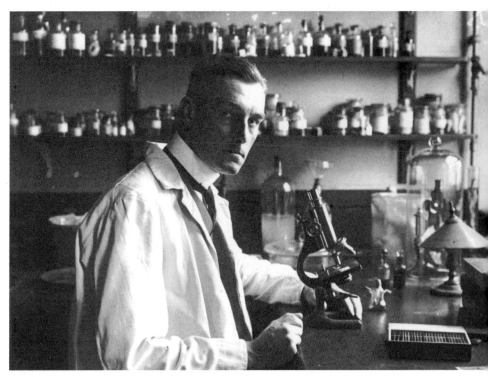

Bernard Spilsbury, the father of modern forensics and devastating expert witness

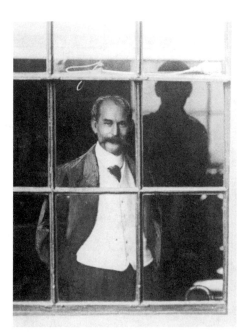

Frederick Seddon, the freemason whose arrogance was almost as shocking as his callousness

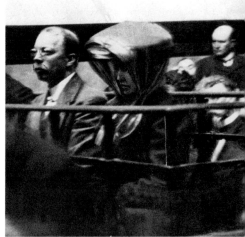

Dr Hawley Harvey Crippen and his mistress Ethel le Neve shortly before Crippen's trial for the murder of his wife, Cora. The forensic evidence would be a vital element

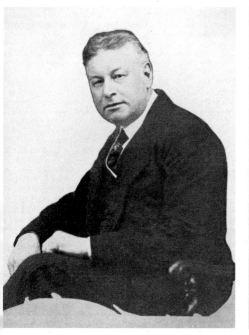

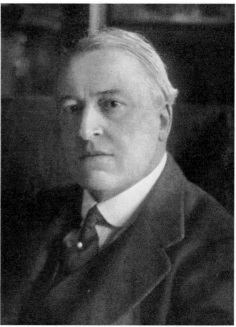

Detective Inspector Arthur Neil of Kentish Town police station. He was 'dogged, determined and a master of careful preparation'

Edward Marshall Hall, the 'Great Defender' who was 'endowed with pre-eminent personal beauty of the most virile type'

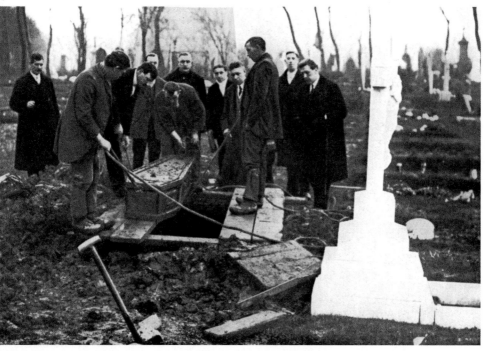

The reinterment of Alice's coffin in Blackpool cemetery. Arthur Neil is standing at the foot of the grave near the gravedigger, and Sergeant Harold Reed is behind on the right with an umbrella on his arm

Bernard Spilsbury's case cards

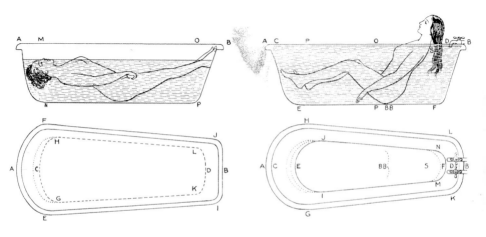

The Herne Bay bath   The Blackpool bath

George Smith: 'Women came journeys of fifty or sixty miles to catch a glimpse of him'

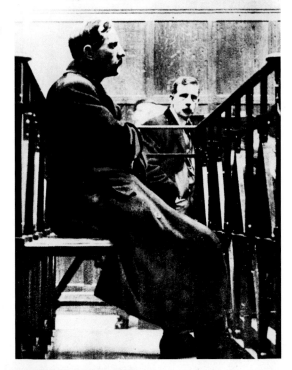

Crowds gathered outside the Old Bailey awaiting developments in the case of the Brides in the Bath

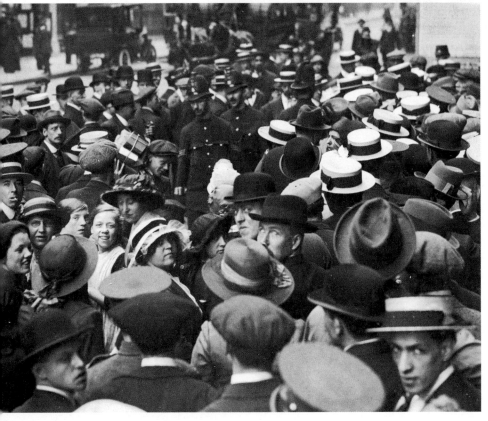

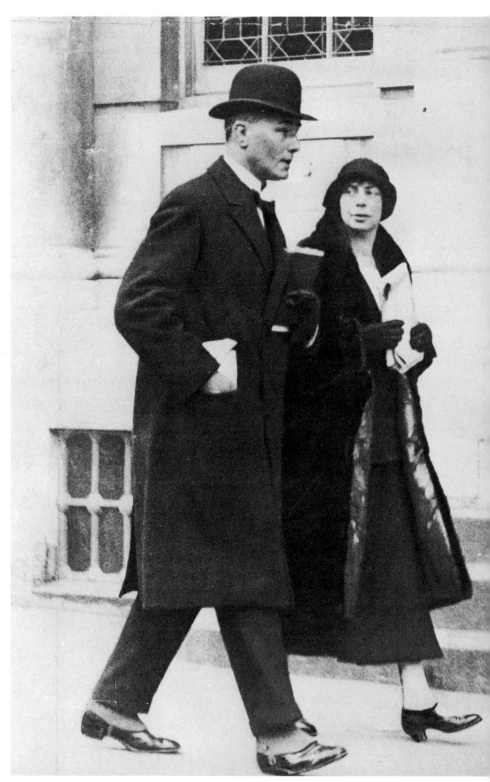

Sir Bernard Spilsbury and his assistant Miss Bainbridge arriving at a murder trial in 1925. He was, by now, perceived as 'the real-life Sherlock Holmes'

it this way – I have a splendid home there awaiting you if you
will forgive me. Do come to Halifax soon as possible there will
be no more obstacles in our way then and you will be the hap-
piest woman in the world. I have great business there to attend
to and must go or I loose my fortune for ever. I have placed
certain money in your luggage and directed it to your home at
Woolwich where you came from – you will find it there for
you . . . Cheer up all is well that ends well.

C. James, The Avenue, Halifax, every one knows me there.
If you love me come soon. Charles x x x

Alice did not see her money again, and Charles had also taken
all her clothes and jewellery. As a result of meeting him, she said,
'I was left with only a few shillings and the clothes I was actually
wearing. What he had taken consisted of the whole of my life's
savings.' Now, on recognizing George Smith, she imagined that
though she had lost all her possessions, it could have been worse:
she might have lost her life.

Alice Reavil's statement raised as many questions as it solved.
If George Smith was, as Inspector Neil suspected, a serial murderer – why did he spare Alice? His marriage to her was
sandwiched between those to Alice Burnham and Margaret
Lofty, both of whom ended up dead. Neil couldn't begin to
comprehend the mind of a man like George Smith, but if he
took pleasure from killing women, why not kill Alice Reavil?
And if he were motivated purely by money, the profits of murder
far outweighed those gained from the cruel little scam that was
marriage followed by desertion. And, for this scam, why was
marriage necessary anyway? A conman might gain a woman's
trust without marrying her. Perhaps this predator felt he had to
dominate a woman through sex, taking her body as a precursor
to taking all her money and belongings. The Inspector knew
that, in terms of understanding his man, his investigation had
scarcely begun. So he dispatched his colleague Detective Inspector
Cole to Somerset House to root around in the records and

discover what he could about George. At the same time a fingerprint search was begun.

The investigations soon turned up a golden nugget of information, the breakthrough that Inspector Neil had been waiting for. As long ago as 1898 George Smith, using the name George Oliver Love, had married a girl named Caroline Thornhill in Leicester. He had given his age as 25; she had been 19. On their marriage certificate, his stated profession was baker and confectioner, hers bootmaker. This woman, thought the Inspector, might well have been Smith's first real wife. Perhaps she would be able to tell the police who he really was, and help them piece together the puzzle of his life. Caroline Thornhill was, he believed, vital to his investigation. But when he asked his officers to track her down, the answer came that she had emigrated to Canada. Inspector Neil wrote to the Canadian Mounted Police asking them to search for her and to persuade her to come to Britain. This was no small request. The Germans had started 'unrestricted submarine warfare', and German U-boats in the Atlantic were torpedoing and sinking around ten ships a week with immense loss of life. Most of the targets were merchant ships carrying cargo to and from Europe, but it was only a matter of time before a passenger liner was struck. Even if Caroline Thornhill were found in Canada, she might easily decide against making such a treacherous journey.

In the meantime, Inspector Neil contacted Bernard Spilsbury and made arrangements for the two men to travel to Herne Bay for the exhumation of Bessie's body, which would happen at dead of night on Friday 19 February. The process was not an easy one – partly because packs of newspaper reporters were following Neil and Spilsbury everywhere, but mainly due to the wartime transformation of the holiday town of Herne Bay. It was now of military importance, thanks to its situation near the port of Dover and close to the mouth of the Thames. In December,

German submarines had tried to enter Dover harbour to torpedo the battleships there, and on Christmas Eve Dover town had been the target for the first enemy bomb ever to be dropped on Britain from the air. It did little damage other than sending a few cabbages flying in a kitchen garden and causing a gardener to fall out of a tree; but the incident served as a warning of future raids.

By February 1915 lookouts were stationed all along the east Kent coast, and strict rules were enforced banning the use of lights at night. Arthur Neil arrived in Herne Bay at dusk, and by the time he reached the graveyard he found that:

> All around the place was barbed wire and fortifications of every description, and our journey to the particular shed where the examination was to take place was made extremely difficult in the dark . . . The military authorities were very touchy at this period about lights of any description owing to the hostile enemy aircraft that visited London via the mouth of the Thames. The sexton was working with a boy on the job, their labour being carried out in pitch darkness. They had commenced work before darkness set in, and by the time we came on the scene they had reached the coffin.

Bessie's grave had become waterlogged, making it difficult to lift the coffin out. Neil found himself straddling the grave, pulling at it 'with my whole might'. It suddenly came free, and he almost fell into the watery pit below. Together with the sextons, he heaved the coffin on to a cart so that it could be wheeled into the town. At the shed that was serving as a mortuary the Williams' neighbour, Percy Millgate, arrived. He had last seen Bessie the day before she died in July 1912, 'when she took a loaf of bread from me'. Now he identified her only by her hair and black eyebrows and the shape of her face. 'When she was alive, her face was round, and very healthy looking', he said. 'She was a tall, well-built woman.'

Bernard Spilsbury's case-card for the post-mortem makes

difficult reading. Bessie's body had been in the ground for two and a half years, and a half-inch opening in the coffin lid had allowed water to leak in. The hair was still firmly attached to the scalp, but the head came away from the body when moved; softer tissues had gone completely: there were no lungs, the liver was shrunken, as were the kidneys and spleen. 'Thick layer sub-cutaneous fat everywhere', Spilsbury wrote, 'and complete adipocere formation.' In this rank fatty slime, he found no evidence of poisoning. Much of the body was wrapped in a shroud that had rotted, ribbed stockings were on the legs and feet and a dark piece of cloth was wrapped around the thighs. When he examined this area closely, he found 'goose skin' – a sort of roughening of the surface that he deemed especially significant.

On his case-card, Spilsbury records Bessie's 'history', as explained by Dr Frank French: his diagnosis of epilepsy; his arrival at 80 High Street; his finding her head under the bath water, and his attempt to resuscitate her. 'Much water drained from mouth, also froth', Spilsbury writes. 'Pressure on stomach expelled more water from mouth – had swallowed water. Face rather blue. Large piece of soap clasped in rt hand. Tongue not bitten. False teeth in mouth. Body was warm.' Spilsbury records the size of Bessie's body and the dimensions of the Herne Bay bath. He also notes that Bessie's husband had been out of the house for half an hour, buying fish. At 8 a.m. when he returned, he 'found her in bath'. Bessie Mundy had drowned, it seemed, shortly before the doctor arrived, and without a struggle.

While Inspector Neil was in Herne Bay, the investigation took a sudden and dramatic new turn. In Bristol a young woman named Edith Pegler had contacted the police to say that she was astounded by the newspaper reports about George Smith. She had instantly recognized him in the press photographs because she had been married to him for the past seven years. Detective Inspector George Cole and Police Sergeant Frank Page dashed to

Paddington station, and took the train to the West Country. At last, the police had someone to interview who knew George Smith intimately, and had known him for years, not just for a few days or weeks.

Edith was a sturdy, plain young woman with a straightforward, no-nonsense air about her. She told officers Cole and Page that she had met George in Bristol 1908 when she answered his advertisement for a domestic servant. At the time, he owned a second-hand furniture shop. 'He engaged me as his housekeeper', she said. 'I had seen him and spoken to him in the shop, but knew nothing of him. After I had been there a week he asked me to marry him. I don't remember if he said much about himself, except that he said he had some money and he wished to settle down. He also said he had an aunt who allowed him money.' They were married on 30 July 1908 at St Peter's register office, Bristol. He gave the name of George Joseph Smith and described himself as a bachelor.

Edith's life with George was unsettled. As soon as they set up a home, he would decide that they should move again. Sometimes they took a second-hand furniture shop, but this never brought in much money. Income, when it materialized, tended to follow George's business trips, which he described as 'going round the country, dealing'. During the early years of their marriage, these trips were fairly short, but they had recently become longer. As a couple, said Edith, they had often returned to Bristol, but they had also lived in Bedford, Luton, Croydon, Southend – where George had bought a house for £270 – East Ham, Walthamstow, Broomhayes, Margate, Tunbridge Wells, Clapham, Cheltenham, Bournemouth, Brighton, Salisbury and Weston-super-Mare. When George bought the house at Southend, he had told Edith that 'he had made this money in connection with a picture he bought and sold at a profit. He said it was a Turner seascape.'

In the summer of 1910, Edith remembered, they had been living at Southend. George had gone away dealing for four or five weeks. 'I had one or two letters from him,' she said, 'and in one of them I remember he mentioned Weymouth.' This was the period in which he had married Bessie and quickly deserted her. When he returned to Edith, 'he said he had been with a young fellow and they had made about £20.'

Early in 1912, George and Edith opened a shop at Bath Road, Brislington, Bristol. 'After we had been there six or seven weeks,' she said:

> he left me saying he was going to have a run round the country again for dealing and was going to try to sell the private house at Southend. He wrote me three or four letters from London at the first part, but after he had been away about five weeks he wrote me telling me to give up the shop and go to Mother's. He finally wrote me about May saying he was going to Canada and would return when he had done some business.

It was during this period – from March to July 1912 – that George was reunited with Bessie in Weston-super-Mare, moved with her to Herne Bay, and left after her death.

His next move was to contact Edith, and persuade her to meet him in Margate. 'He told me he had been to Canada and had made about a £1,000 through dealing. He said he met another young fellow there and they had some things they were going to sell in London.' George, said Edith, had used the money to buy some more houses, this time in Bristol, selling them shortly afterwards at a loss.

In September 1913, said Edith, 'I stayed with my Mother and he left me saying he had lost money on his property and he was going away dealing to see if he could make it up. I heard from him a day or two later from London. He sent me some money – I think £6. He told me to stay at Mother's as he was going to Spain.' It was that September that George met Alice Burnham on the seafront at Southsea.

Edith heard no more from him until the evening of 22

December 1913, when he returned unexpectedly to celebrate Christmas at home. This was ten days after Alice's death.

> He said, he had come from Spain and the young fellow he was with and he were selling jewellery he had bought in Spain. He let me understand that his journey had been profitable. He remained with us over Christmas 1913, but we slept at another house as there was no accommodation at Mother's house.

From Edith's point of view, 1914 was a relatively stable time. While war engulfed Europe, she spent the summer at Bournemouth and Brighton; then she and George took a three-week holiday in Torquay, and invited Edith's mother to join them for a fortnight. On returning from Devon, they moved into rented rooms in Bournemouth. While there George went out every evening, and in the middle of September he left the town, saying he was going to London for a few days. After a week, he sent Edith a postcard saying he would soon be home. This was the period in which George had met Alice Reavil on the seafront at Bournemouth, romanced her every evening, married her, and deserted her in Brockwell Park. 'About a week later,' said Edith, 'I received a letter from him, asking me to go to Weston-super-Mare to an address he gave. I went and he told me he had been to a sale in London and had bought some lady's clothing. He had some left and gave it to me. It was kept in a black trunk which I had not seen before.'

He left home again about three weeks before Christmas 1914, saying he was going to London to do some dealing. Edith went to her mother's house, and heard no more from her husband until 23 December,

> when he casually walked in about 7 or 8 p.m. He remained over Christmas 1914 for about a week. He then left and said he was going to London over a picture for which he could not get the money. He was away about 10 days, and then came back for a week or so. He went away again for a week or so and finally left

on the 1 Feb. 1915 at about 8 a.m. saying he was going to try and get the money for his picture. I have not seen him, nor heard from him since.

This was the period in which George, as John Lloyd, had married Margaret Lofty and in which she had died in the bath.

Edith's statement is infused with her pain and sorrow. Despite his unpredictability, she had loved her husband, and had never had the slightest suspicion that George was marrying other women, let alone murdering them. But when she looked back on it, there were some peculiar aspects to his behaviour. She remembered one time in 1913 when she and George had taken a motor charabanc trip to Wells and Glastonbury. During the journey they fell into conversation with a governess named Florence Hayward, and when they all returned to Weston-super-Mare, George remained friendly with Florence. He told Edith that he thought it might be a good idea for him to take out an insurance policy on Florence's life. He would pay the premiums, regarding them as an investment. 'I did not agree and we had some words,' said Edith. 'I could not see the object of it and said to him "I don't think you can afford to keep up the payments, adding that he might have to keep on paying for 50 years or more".' He said he could afford it and it was just as good an investment as anything else.' Florence came to tea to discuss it, and, according to George, he took out the policy and paid one premium before giving up the idea.

A police enquiry uncovered a slightly different version of events. The insurance company, in reality, had refused the policy. George, the police learned, was 'on affectionate terms' with Florence. 'The girl seems to have become very friendly with one of the insurance people, and this seems to have enraged Smith, who went to her employers, and told them she was a bad girl, and not fit to have the custody of their children.'

On another occasion, this time in 1912 when George was

living with Bessie in Herne Bay, Edith had become exasperated by his long absences. Between March and August that year she tried to reach him. 'I received letters from him from Ramsgate,' she said, 'but bearing no address, and he told me in one that he was going to Canada and should not return until he had made his fortune and he advised me to take a situation.' Instead, Edith took the train from Bristol to London, and then on down to Ramsgate, where she spent six days walking the streets and asking at banks, hoping to find her husband, 'because I was doubtful about him having gone to Canada'. Eventually she gave up and went home, unaware that she had come within a whisker of finding George living with Bessie in Herne Bay. When George found out that she had followed him, 'he was very angry about it and said he should never tell me his business again'. And when Edith had mentioned an annuity that George had purchased, 'he remarked to me that if I interfered with his business I should never have another happy day'.

George was threatening to Edith, but he was sometimes affectionate too. And even though he was often away on his mysterious trips, he always came back – like a bad penny. Sometimes, he was quite the family man – playing the piano for Edith and her mother, making sure he was there at Christmas. He had put Edith in a special category and her life, it seems, had never been in danger. And perhaps Alice Reavil was also a special case. The two women were, in fact, different from the three who died. They were domestic servants, very much of the lower orders, like George himself. But Bessie Mundy, Alice Burnham and Margaret Lofty came from families which were a cut above: the middling classes. George, when he encountered the Burnhams en masse at Aston Clinton demonstrated a deep hostility to all of them, and when Alice died everyone remembered the lie he told. Her relatives would not come to the funeral, he had said, because 'they are too common and too poor'. A hierarchical society in which everyone was expected to know his place

enraged George, and he loathed those who considered themselves his superior. Edith and Alice, as domestic servants, could
not be so presumptuous.

The police, of course, hoped that Edith would be able to provide them with incriminating evidence. Did he, they asked, have
any special interest in poisons? Drugs, they thought, might have
been given to his doomed wives to produce the peculiar headaches that had come on just before they died. And perhaps drugs
had rendered these women supine and ready to acquiesce to his
wishes. But Edith said her husband had no interest in drugs
or poisons. In fact, 'the only medicine he took was Epsom Salts,
which he took frequently and he always kept a supply'. And he
had never suggested to Edith that she insure her life, or make a
will in his favour. 'If I am insured,' she said, 'I am not aware
of it.'

As for baths:

> I have never known him enquire at any of the apartments we
> have been to for a bath, as he remarked to me on more than one
> occasion that he did not believe in using baths in apartment
> houses, which other people had access to. I remember once at
> Weston-super-Mare he had a bath, but all the time I have
> known him this is the only time he has had a bath in a bathroom
> to my knowledge.

She did remember, though, that just after Christmas in 1914,
when they were living in apartments in Bristol, Edith had told
George that she was going to have a bath. He said, 'In that bath
there? [referring to the bathroom] I should advise you to be careful of those things as it is known that women often lost their lives
through weak hearts and fainting in a bath.'

On 26 February another young woman came forward. Arthur
Neil took her statement. Her name, she said, was Flora Walter
and she had met George Smith on the front at Brighton in June

1908. She had been sitting with a friend, when he came and sat next to them. 'He spoke to us, and remarked about the weather and from that we got into conversation. He said that he was a man of means . . . He had, he said, been a carpenter and was now a dealer in antiques. He saw us off from Brighton that evening by train and made arrangements to come over to Worthing to see me the next day. I was then in business at an Art Needlework shop at Worthing. In the course of the conversation, I told him I was a widow.'

After a few days George proposed to Flora. She accepted him and gave up her job. 'In the course of some conversation with me,' she said, 'he asked if I was insured, and although I was, I told him that I was not.' Her lie suggests that she did not trust him totally, an unease that was intensified when George asked Flora 'what amount of money I had, and all about myself. He insisted on seeing my Bank Book and I showed it to him. The amount was £33 13s 0d.' George suggested that they go to London, and on 3 July 1908 the couple visited the post office in Camden Town so that Flora could draw out all her money. Before she knew it, George had taken the cash, saying he would look after it.

When they left the post office, George said, 'Come along dear,' and suggested they visit the Franco-British exhibition in Shepherd's Bush. It cost a shilling to enter, so was a relatively cheap day out. But the couple had been at the exhibition only five minutes, said Flora, 'when he left me sitting on a seat saying that he was going to get a paper and would be back in a few minutes.' She waited about half an hour on the bench, and when he didn't show up she realized that she had been right to be suspicious. She hesitated no longer, and found a police constable.

With a police escort, Flora returned to their rented rooms in Chelsea, and then to the cloakroom at Victoria station where she had left her belongings. George had taken everything, even her clothes. 'The total value of my property, together with the money which Smith took, amounted to about £80 to £90' – more than a yea 's salary at the needlework shop.

This was the earliest example to come to light of George's criminal exploitation of the single women that he met. But Arthur Neil suspected that his abuse of his girlfriends and wives had a much longer history, and that Caroline Thornhill, the 'first wife' who had emigrated to Canada, knew more about George than anyone else. It was frustrating that she had disappeared to the other side of the world but not, in the light of George's heinous behaviour, very surprising. Perhaps she had decided that she would feel safe only if separated from her husband by the vastness of the Atlantic Ocean. And even then, it was quite possible that George's endless fantasizing about Canada was based in reality, and that he had gone there, trying to find her. There were, after all, many years of his adult life that were so far unaccounted for, and unexplained. Throughout the investigations, the prisoner himself said little – and the information he did give generally turned out to be a lie.

The weeks passed with no news from Canada, and then in early March the Inspector received a letter from the Inspector of Police in Saskatoon saying that Caroline had been found. 'I have the honour to report,' he wrote, 'that this woman is now living near Asquith under the name of Mrs George Bowness, and has positively identified herself as the party wanted in England. She is quite willing to return to England and give evidence against her husband.' He asked for her steamship fare and other expenses to be forwarded, including $15 cash for incidentals, since 'this woman has absolutely no money'. Evidently, Caroline Thornhill was a brave woman with a story to tell. Scotland Yard paid up, and she began the long, perilous journey home. On 30 March, her ship, the SS *Corsican*, docked at Liverpool. The voyage had been without incident, but Caroline had been lucky. A few weeks later, on 7 May, a German U-boat torpedoed the Cunard liner the *Lusitania* when she was close to the Irish coast. The ship sank in just eighteen minutes and 1,198 of the 1,959 passengers were drowned.

As Caroline came down the gangplank, the British press was at the ready. The next day's papers revealed that 'Mrs Bowness' seemed no longer to be a married woman, and she was met in Liverpool by a fine-looking Canadian soldier who embraced her warmly. On the same day, she was interviewed by Detective Inspector George Cole.

Finally, a clearer picture of George Smith's background emerged. Caroline had met him in Leicester in 1897, she said, and he had told her of a difficult childhood. He had grown up in Bethnal Green in London's East End. He had started thieving as a young boy, and been sent away to a Reform School at the age of 9 – where he stayed until he was 16 (his mother had said 'that boy will die with his boots on'). Although George was a compulsive liar, this particular tale has a ring of truth about it. He had told Caroline his school had been at Gravesend, on the Thames, midway between Herne Bay and London – and the Milton Industrial School that was in Gravesend at the time was, indeed, filled with boys like George. Described as a 'damp old country mansion in a state of depression', it was a legacy of the Victorians' mission to cure 'juvenile depravity'.

There, George would have found himself with other boys from the lower classes. Some were juvenile offenders, others were simply outcasts and guilty of nothing other than being poor. Such schools were populated by children 'who are found begging or wandering, or are the children of tramps and ne'er-do-weels, who have no proper guardianship provided for them'. Many were 'taken from immoral surroundings', or removed from home for being beyond the control of their parents, or for persistent truanting.

Life at the Industrial School was harsh, and could be expected to give anyone a sense of grievance. Social rejection and public humiliation were at its heart, and the authorities ensured that pupils stood out from other children because of their ugly, badly fitting uniforms and closely cropped hair. 'It is not an uncommon sight, in some towns', wrote the reformer Mary Barnett in 1913, 'to see the local Industrial or Reformatory School marching through the streets for all the world as if they were young convicts'.

At the great majority of schools money was used as the principal incentive for encouraging good work – boys being given a few pence each week in return for any good marks in their studies. Bad behaviour was often punished with a thrashing – sometimes in front of the whole school. For the most serious offences, such as trying to abscond or 'malingering', Barnett observed, 'a cane or a birch is used, a maximum of twelve strokes being allowed in the Industrial Schools and of eighteen in the Reformatories'. Very little attention, she said, was given to reading – but a great deal to sport and military drilling. Boys who graduated from such schools often joined the army or the navy. At George's school, the main subjects on the curriculum were carpentry, book-making, tailoring, farm work, laundry work and baking.

By 1897 George, now 25 years old and calling himself 'George Love', was in Leicester where he bought a bakery business. Caroline Thornhill, aged 18, came to work for him, and before long they became sweethearts. George asked Caroline to marry him and, when she accepted, he, in the proper way, went to see her parents to ask for her hand. But Mr and Mrs Thornhill disliked Caroline's choice of husband and objected to the marriage. Caroline had always been close to her family. Nonetheless, she decided to go ahead without their consent, and George arranged a wedding at St Matthew's Church. Arthur Elliott, the sexton there, remembered it well seventeen years later, because, he said, 'Love made so much fuss about it.' Elliott thought that George wanted a fancy occasion in order to impress the local people who might buy bread from his shop. Caroline's parents didn't come, but her father watched from a distance as she went into the church.

Two years later, Caroline was in Lewes prison awaiting trial for a theft in Hastings, on the south coast. It was her husband, she said, who had made her do it. He had now deserted her, and she gave the police a statement that might help them find him and bring him to justice. His description, she said, is 'complexion fair, hair brown, ginger moustache, when he left me he was growing sideboards, peak chin, left arm a very large scar, military walk, stands five feet nine inches'. He had a background of thieving: 'On one occasion he stole some money from an aunt, and a bicycle, and was sent to prison for six months.'

She was unsure of his real name. 'Some of his people call him Joe Smith,' she said, 'and some of his friends call him George Oliver Love. He went into the army as Smith.' George had told her that he had served three years in the Northamptonshire Regiment, until he received a discharge for bad conduct. When he left, he took up with a woman at the Elephant and Castle, then forced her take a job as a domestic servant and bullied her into stealing from her employers. It was while George was pawning a stolen watch in the Strand that he 'got caught and was took to Bow Street and from there to Chelsea, and got twelve months . . . He done it at Wormwood Scrubs. I do not know what name it was in, but I think it was Wilson.'

On leaving prison he once again persuaded the woman to steal for him. When she came home, one day, with a cash-box containing £115, he took the money, and went to Leicester, where he opened the bakery at Russell Square.

After the Leicester bakery business failed, said Caroline, 'he did no work and his money began to get short and he suggested that I should go into service with references supplied by him and steal from the people'. When she objected, 'he abused me and threatened me,' so that after a time she gave in. She took five or six jobs in London, using the different names that George suggested for her, and stole jewellery from her employers. George 'would be waiting outside the house for me to bring it out and then we would go to Islington and he would make me pledge it. He would never pledge it himself. He always told me how much to ask for it. Some of it was sold to a Receiver in Islington.'

George had decided that it was wise to be on the move. The couple went from London to Croydon to Birmingham, and on to Hove where Caroline stole from a clergyman's house. 'We then went to Hastings and I went into a situation there and stole some property. He went with me to pledge this property and waited outside . . . I was arrested and he ran away.'

Caroline served a three-month prison sentence, and when she left started a new life as a domestic servant working for a Detective Inspector Arrow. A year later, on 5 November 1900, she said, she was in Oxford Street in London when she saw George looking in the window of a shop. She approached two policemen and George was taken into custody. 'He abused me very much and said he would punch my head off if he could only get at me. He accused me of being an immoral woman and was very violent and tried to get away from the policemen to get at me.' Caroline and her mother went to Hastings for George's subsequent trial, and gave evidence against him. On 9 January 1901 he was sentenced to two years in prison.

Caroline returned to Leicester and took a job in a shoe factory. In early 1903 she heard that George was out of prison and had come looking for her. One day she came home and saw him waiting outside her house. 'I don't think he saw me. My two brothers went after him and gave him a thrashing and since then I have never seen him, nor heard from him. I went to Canada on 31 May 1906, and have lived there ever since.'

A month after Caroline gave her statement another woman came forward to tell her story. Sarah Falkner said that in June 1909 (a year after George married Edith) she met a man named George Rose in Southampton. They fell into conversation 'with the result that I finally went for a walk with him'. In the following days George called regularly at the lodging house where Sarah rented a room, and took her for walks. After a fortnight he asked her to marry him. At first she refused him, but he 'told me he would follow me up till I did marry him' and finally she relented. 'He said he had money in the Bank, but I never saw any evidence of it.' They were married on the morning of 29 October 1909 at Southampton register office. After the little ceremony George and Sarah returned to her lodgings, picked up her belongings, and took the 11.15 a.m. train to Clapham Junction.

George, said Sarah, persuaded her to withdraw all her savings from the post office, so that he could open a business as an antique dealer. She had, she said, £260 in cash and £30 in government stock. Her new husband accompanied her to Lavender Hill post office and picked up all the money as the assistant handed it over. 'I asked him for some of it,' said Sarah, 'but he would not give me any.'

> After we left the Post Office we went to the National Picture Gallery and while there he asked me to excuse him and asked me to sit down . . . I waited an hour and then went and made some enquiry but could not find him. I therefore went back to the lodgings. On looking into my bag I found all my money gone with the exception of a few pence . . .

George Rose, she said, 'left me penniless – with the exception of the few coppers mentioned – and I had to borrow to pay the lodgings.' He took all her jewellery, and left nothing behind other than three empty boxes. She thought that, in total, he had robbed her of £400.

'I have seen George Joseph Smith', she told officers Cole and Page, 'and he is identical with George Rose, and he is the man I married . . . I have not my marriage certificate as he took it away with him.' Sarah, like George's other victims, was a young woman of modest means, who had managed to put much of her income into a savings account. She didn't ask a lot from life, but had hoped for a romance and a husband.

In his report of 18 May 1915, Arthur Neil wrote. 'this brings the number of marriages contracted by the prisoner since 1898 to seven, three of the women having died whilst taking a bath'. The police investigation before the magistrate, he continued, had so far necessitated calling 121 witnesses against Smith.

8

Drowning

Drowning is an unusual form of murder in life, and in literature. Maybe this is because people assume that it is hard to drown someone without a struggle – without the victim thrashing about, fighting back. A struggle attracts attention and raises the possibility of escape. It is risky. And drowning is, it's commonly thought, also arduous. The murderer who chooses drowning is relying on his own brute strength, and on the weakness of his victim, unlike the killer who stabs or shoots or poisons.

The murder at the heart of Emile Zola's novel, *Thérèse Raquin,* is this type of drowning – loud, messy and violent. It starts in a boat on the river, with a struggle between Thérèse's lover, Laurent, and her husband Camille, as she watches on in silence. Laurent, wrote Zola,

> bent his head and exposed his neck, his victim, mad with rage and terror, twisted himself, lowered his head and dug his teeth into Laurent's neck. And when the murderer, repressing a cry of pain, suddenly threw the clerk into the river, Camille's teeth tore off a piece of Laurent's flesh. He fell in shrieking. He came to the surface two or three times, shouting more and more weakly.

So that passers-by will not be suspicious, Laurent capsizes the boat, and pretends there has been an accident.

Once dead, Camille's body gives away no clues – and that is the advantage of a drowning. No bullet holes, no knife wounds, no residual poison. Zola's description of it is informed by the novelist's visits to the Paris morgue, and his inspection of drowned corpses. Like Bernard Spilsbury, he has been close to the bodies of the dead and tried to understand them; his description reads like a Spilsbury case-card, only with all the revulsion that a scientist must exclude, left in:

> the eyelids raised showing the pale globes of the eyeballs; the twisted lips, pulled to one side of the mouth, were set in a hideous grin; the tip of the blackened tongue showed between the white teeth . . . the body seemed to be a pile of dissolved flesh; it had suffered horribly from the water. One could tell that the arms were no longer attached; the clavicle bones were sticking through the skin of the shoulders. The ribs made black stripes on the greenish chest; the left side, which had burst open, was only a jumble of dark red tatters. The whole body was rotting. The legs, which were better preserved, were stretched out and covered with revolting blotches. The feet were falling off.

Forensic science had no role to play in the story that followed. In terms of criminal detection, this was a drowned body, and that was that. And the pathologist had no role to play in the cases of killing by drowning that appeared in the British newspapers in the early part of the twentieth century. These were overwhelmingly of one type – mothers drowning their babies and small children. In 1904 Maria Martin of Lambeth drowned her three young children, the eldest of them being just four and a half years. In 1905 Louisa Pole drowned her two daughters, 8-year-old Elsie and 7-year-old Kate, in the bath-tub. In 1909 Edith Baldock drowned her three children in the bath – the eldest of whom was 6, and the youngest 18 months. In each case the mother was found to be not responsible for her actions. Louisa Pole had suffered from melancholia, and was said to be in a 'state often found among the insane after a mental explosion'. Edith Baldock, said the coroner, was suffering from 'some sort of temporary insanity'. All three distraught mothers confessed to their actions. Of all the 259 judicial hangings in Britain in the years 1900–14, only three are for murder by drowning – each of them a man convicted of drowning small children. Drowning an adult might be a risky business, but drowning a child was, from the physical perspective, manageable. And in *Thérèse Raquin*, Camille is sickly and as weak as a child.

One case of adult drowning does, however, stand out. In December 1912 the tabloid press became excited by a death in the sea near Newquay in Cornwall. Mrs Marian Nowill had been staying at the Atlantic Hotel, and after a cliff-top walk had somehow ended up in the ocean below. It was strongly implied in the press that a fellow guest at the hotel, Mr Delay, was her lover. Mr Delay was found hanged in his room on the day that Mrs Nowill vanished from the cliff-top. Had he pushed her over the edge, and then taken his own life? To illustrate the story, the newspapers published a snapshot of Mrs Nowill sitting in a deckchair on the beach, wearing fashionable clothes and a smart hat. On her left was her husband, who was slightly tubby and bore a vague resemblance to the late King Edward VII, while Mr Delay, in the deckchair to her right, was more dashing and handsome. The Nowills had met Mr Delay, the papers reported, on a P&O cruise.

The coroner heard evidence from Mrs Nowill's husband Sidney, who described his wife as a supremely honourable woman who would never have contemplated an affair with Mr Delay. The jury was then asked to consider how Mrs Nowill had met her death – she might have been walking on the cliffs, said the coroner, and fallen in accidentally; she might have thrown herself into the water and committed suicide; or she might have been forced or thrown in the water by someone else.

Forensic science, on this occasion, did play a part. The doctor who performed the post-mortem said there were no signs of violence on the body. She apparently went into the water living, and died from asphyxia caused by drowning. He noticed a 'slight mottling of the lungs', which, he said, showed that she had made very little effort to save herself. 'It is not a mathematical certainty,' he added, 'but it is said that the more struggling there is, the more mottling takes place. In this case there was very little mottling.' So, he was suggesting, a struggle did not simply raise the risk of alerting witnesses – it also left a detectable trace upon the body.

In the end, the way in which Mrs Nowill found her way into the sea remained a mystery. The coroner said: 'There was not a shadow of a doubt that Delay had behaved in the most heartless and cruel way to this poor woman.' But beyond that, the jury could not go. A verdict was returned of 'found drowned'.

Few cases of drowning came Bernard Spilsbury's way. But there was, in his world, a scholarly interest in the subject, and in October 1909 the Medico-Legal Society, in which he played a prominent part, hosted a lecture on drowning.

The talk was given by F. G. Crookshank, the police surgeon to the Thames Division of the Metropolitan Police, whose daily life concerned the examination of bodies fished out of the river. 'When a living person enters the water and death occurs,' he said, 'there is often of course a struggle and submersion alternating with appearance at the surface. In such cases death is due to asphyxia from drowning.' But sometimes, he said, the person sinks and dies without a struggle. This could be due to a pre-existing condition, such as epilepsy or syncope (a heart condition). Often it is due to 'inhibition' – a sort of sudden shock.

To explain his idea of 'inhibition', he told the story of a woman who jumped off Waterloo Bridge 'one foggy night'. Several hours later her body was found up-river at Barnes. Her death, he said, was due to inhibition – the shock caused when she went into the water so suddenly. Death from 'inhibition' was much faster than conventional drowning and occurs, he said, 'when functions are arrested by excitation of a distant part of the nervous system'. It is 'a reflex through the medulla, and causes death calmly without a struggle . . . Death appears to be sudden. Death is mechanical rather than chemical.' He thought that 'inhibition' was responsible for about one-third of the deaths by drowning in the Thames.

Bernard Spilsbury's colleague, William Willcox, participated in the discussion that followed. He was interested to learn, he said, that so many people had met their deaths in the Thames, 'not by drowning but by other causes. It was too often assumed that when a dead body was found in the water the death was due to drowning.' He was 'greatly interested' in the importance that Crookshank attached to 'inhibition'.

In the summer of 1914, when war broke out, Bernard Spilsbury decided to take his family on holiday to Bude, in north Cornwall. He took with him a copy of a popular book, published in 1903, called *Footprints of Former Men in Far Cornwall*. The author was the Revd Robert S. Hawker, who had been Vicar of Morwenstow, a village by the sea, just north of Bude. Hawker's prose is lively and full of drama (some said he was reluctant to let the facts get in the way of a good story), particularly in the account he gives of the drowning of the crew of the *Caledonia*, a Scottish ship that was wrecked off the Cornish coast in 1842. 'About daybreak of an Autumn day, I was aroused by a knock at the bedroom door; it was followed by the agitated voice of a boy, a member of my household, "Oh sir, there are dead men on the vicarage rocks!"' Hawker was out of bed in an instant, put on his dressing-gown, and rushed across the cliffs to the shore, where he found two dead sailors, 'stiff and stark'. 'The bay was tossing and seething with a tangled mass of rigging, sails and broken fragments of a ship; the billows rolled up yellow with corn, for the cargo of the vessel had been foreign wheat.'

Bodies were everywhere, some under rocks

jammed in by the force of the water, so that it took sometimes several ebb-tides, and the strength of many hands, to extricate the corpses. The captain I came upon myself lying placidly upon his back, with his arms folded . . . The hand of the spoiler was about to assail him when I suddenly appeared, so that I rescued him untouched. Each hand grasped a small pouch or bag. One contained his pistols; the other held two little log-reckoners of brass.

The fact that the captain had objects clenched in his hands at the moment of his death, as Bessie Mundy had clasped the soap as she drowned, was seen as evidence of a very sudden end.

During his holiday, Spilsbury boated and fished, and read this book. On the fly-leaf, under the heading 'Medico-Legal notes', he wrote several comments, one of which was 'p. 60 – retention of articles in the hands of shipwrecked men'. Perhaps the soap in Bessie's hand was evidence that she died extremely quickly – like the woman who threw herself off Waterloo Bridge, and the captain who was dashed on the Cornish rocks, maybe in a way that Crookshank would have called 'inhibition'. Bernard Spilsbury took the view that this – or something like it – was the case, that Bessie's death had been immediate, that she had no chance to come up for air. She was a big woman, and her death in a bath was quite unlike those of the poor children drowned by their mothers or, in fiction, of Camille who succumbed, after a fight, because he was frail. He now had the ingenious idea of testing out the theory of a quick death, and asked Inspector Neil to set up an experiment.

Neil duly arranged for the three baths, from Herne Bay, Blackpool and Highgate, to be brought to his police station in Kentish Town. 'Bernard Spilsbury and I had gone over the measurement of each one, over and over again,' he wrote. 'His measurements of each woman were carefully calculated and taken into consideration, kneeling, sitting and lying positions all being gone into and carefully thought out by him and William Willcox. The smallest bath of the three was the Blackpool one, very little difference arising between the other two.' His mission was

to make some demonstration in the baths with women of a similar stature to the dead brides. This was arrived at by minute questioning of their relatives about these women in life – also from Bernard Spilsbury's measurements and weights. The motive being for the purpose of ascertaining the displacement of water before – and after – the bodies were in the baths. For this purpose I obtained the assistance of a very fine lady swimmer, and one used to diving, plunging and swimming from early girlhood. The baths were filled up and in each one demonstrations were given by this young lady in a swimming costume in many positions.

Two demonstrations took place with the young lady swimmer, one in the bath at full length, pressed down by the forehead. In this position, although helpless, the arms can be thrown out to clutch the sides of the bath. Nevertheless, a strong pressure upon the forehead would occasion suffocation and insensibility within a few seconds. On the other hand, a demonstration by myself and sergeants on her, nearly proved fatal.

It was decided to test sudden immersion, so, from the ankle I lifted up her legs very suddenly. She slipped under easily, but to me, who was closely watching, she seemed to make no movement.

Suddenly I gripped her arm, it was limp. With a shout I tugged at her arm-pit and raised her head above the water. It fell over to one side. She was unconscious. For nearly half an hour my detectives and I worked away at her with artificial respiration and restoratives. Things began to look serious, and then a quick change began to take place, and her pretty face began to take on the natural bloom of young healthy womanhood. It had given us all a turn, so practical demonstrations in baths were from that moment promptly discontinued. She told us afterwards that immediately she went under the water with her legs held in the air, the water just rushed into her mouth and up her nostrils. That was all she knew, as she remembered no more until she came to and saw all our anxious faces bending over.

This, at last, seemed a credible theory to explain the speed and ease with which George seemed to have drowned his victims. He had, thought Neil and Spilsbury, whipped up his wives' legs, and they had shot into the water so quickly that death happened almost instantaneously.

Members of the public sent in other ideas. John Lambert of Shrewsbury Road, Redhill, Surrey, wrote in to describe a murder that he had read about in a detective story in a monthly magazine. The killer, he wrote, had pierced the brain of his victim with a long curved needle inserted into the skull through the eye socket.

> May I ask if this is practical? and could this story have any bearing on the present cases? Did it aid the crime? . . . Did the [bath] water contain any evidence? Did drowning only *follow* death? Has the defendant studied medicine or surgery, more or less?'
> . . . I have no knowledge of the defendant beyond that aroused by the press and the ordinary desire to see justice done.

Captain Morgan of the Royal Artillery Mess, Aldershot, suggested that since there was no evidence of violence or poison, it might be worth investigating whether George had actually electrocuted his wives in their baths. Mr F. Marchant of Highgate, a member of the Institution of Civil Engineers, had another idea:

> It is quite possible to suffocate a person recumbent in a bath by pouring into it a sufficiency of carbonic acid gas. This gas is easily made, can be poured from one vessel to another like water, it being very much heavier than air. Lots of lives have been lost by it accidentally in well-sinking, sewers and other places. It is the gaseous element in aerated waters. Such suffoca-

tion would leave no trace capable of detection by chemical analysis.

The letter was passed by the DPP to William Willcox, because of his expertise in toxicology, who replied that the suggestion was 'not applicable in the current case'. He had, himself, received several other theories, he said, none of which were relevant.

The question of how George Smith might have drowned women in their baths with nobody noticing inevitably went beyond the mechanics of the situation and explored the psychology. Mr Fred Heaven of Scarborough wrote in:

> The question naturally arises why Miss Mundy neither called out nor shouted when she was being murdered – and my suggestion is that she was under the impression that her husband was pulling her about in fun and play and that he kept up this illusion – probably by laughing and joking quietly until she was too weak and exhausted to defend herself – he in the meantime pulling and pushing her body about violently until his purpose was attained. She would naturally in her nude state and believing he was only playing with her hesitate to bring anyone to the scene, and she may even have died believing he was playing with her. The prisoner has proved himself a past master in the art of cunning and deceit and may well have kept his victim under this illusion to the end.

Mr M. Ohma of the London Vaudeville Agency also wrote: 'No doubt you will have heard of me in consequence of my success in America and this country, which I have achieved in my practice as a Hypnotist.' He had, he said, 'carefully studied the portrait of the accused Smith, as it appeared in the Press', and had reached the 'unshakeable conclusion' that Smith possessed hypnotic powers: 'These poor women have met their fate while under that influence . . . I shall be delighted to call upon you' he continued, 'to . . . discuss with you a plan, by means of which I might get a statement from the accused himself, that he is a hyp-notist'. Mr Ohma's proposal was noted by the office of the Director of Public Prosecutions, then politely turned down.

The writer Eric Watson consulted both Inspector Neil and Bernard Spilsbury for a long essay considering how it was that George Smith had such power. How did he impose his will so absolutely on three different women, 'each coming from a home superior to his, and each boasting a greater degree of education'? The impression he made was so absolute that each 'surrendered all to him that they had in the world – their bodies and their belongings with equal abandon'.

It was all to do, he wrote, with the psychology of sex and the ability of two radically different types of men to impress women. The first, he said, possessed a 'marked femininity of character', allowing him to understand women from their own point of view. The second was of a 'very pronounced masculinity'. This man's success 'is due to the arousing of women's primitive desire to be mastered'. George Smith took such mastery to an abnor-mal, sadistic level, using all the instincts of a 'lady's man'. His antennae told him in an instant which of the women he met might succumb to his dubious charms, and who would be repelled.

Physical attractiveness was a part of the equation. George, said Watson, had 'a certain magnetism about his eyes', that drew women to him. One of his conquests spoke of his 'extraordinary power over women. This power lay in his eyes. When he looked at you for a minute or two you had the feeling that you were being magnetised. They were little eyes that seemed to rob you of your will.'

Some who met George Smith suggested that he did, indeed, as the Vaudeville artist Mr Ohma had believed, have hypnotic powers; and Watson considered the possibility seriously. In 1894 George du Maurier had published the best-selling novel *Trilby*, in which his hypnotist, the infamous Svengali, 'by mesmeric art, compels the surrender of the heroine to his revolting person'. Was it possible that Bessie, Alice and Margaret were persuaded by similar powers to submit to Smith: to marry him, make wills and take out insurance policies in his favour? George Witzoff, the 'arch bigamist' of 1905, had been a hypnotist. The newspapers reported that Witzoff, an American, had gained power over a hundred women, persuading them to marry him by using 'the silent Hindoo method' of hypnosis. He robbed each of his wives of her modest life savings, before moving on to the next. Photographs showed him, dressed up in a turban and a long robe, his arms outstretched and lines of light emanating from hands that hovered over the face of a swooning woman. His penetrating eyes were staring darkly. Now, ten years later, the memory of Witzoff was resurrected in reports of Smith's unnatural influence over women. Only after Witzoff, commented the *Weekly Dispatch*, did George Smith appear to come up with a 'professional bridegroom plan'.

The expert, H. E. Wingfield, wrote in 1910 that a successful hypnotist should have a commanding tone to his voice, should repeat his message forcefully, and should have a powerful personality. George's letters reveal him as a master at driving home a command (the letter in which he instructs Bessie to tell her relatives that she has 'lost' her money is the most striking example), endlessly repeating the fine detail of the instructions, and his forcefulness was not in question. The idea seemed reasonable, but in the end Watson dismissed hypnosis in favour of a theory rooted in the general psychology of the female sex.

Women were, he thought, actually attracted by George's depravity and by his aggressive sexuality; and the sort of woman who was susceptible might look quite ordinary on the outside. He quotes the famous sexologist, Havelock Ellis: 'nowhere does the trained observer meet with more sensual women than are to be found in quiet homes and country vicarages'. To the common eye a young woman who worships at the chapel or in her father's church may seem innocent and demure. But in secret 'she is also a worshipper of the pagan divinity Priapus'. George Smith, wrote Watson,

> could read very well the mind of a woman, and could see whether in the depths of her eyes could be traced the smoulder-ing fires of passion, all the more ready to burst into flame from the constant repression of desire forced on her by the daily round and common task, be it governess or lady's companion, or young lady in business.

A woman's desire to surrender herself to a man was, despite the suffragette movement, commonly accepted. Bernard Spilsbury's colleague at St Mary's, Almroth Wright, argued in *The Times* that the entire future of matrimony depended on 'willing subor-dination on the part of the wife'. It was much discussed in popular magazines (as in *Strand Magazine*'s debate on 'What Sort of Man a Woman Likes') and taken for granted even by Havelock Ellis, a forward-thinking proponent of sexual liberation. It is easy, he believed,

> to trace in women a delight in experiencing physical pain when inflicted by a lover, and an eagerness to accept subjection to his will. Such a tendency is certainly normal. To abandon herself to her lover, to be able to rely on his physical strength and mental resourcefulness, to be swept out of herself and beyond the con-trol of her own will, to drift idly in delicious submission to another and stronger will – this is one of the commonest aspir-ations in a young woman's intimate love-dreams . . .

In these terms, the complete surrender of Bessie, Alice and Margaret to a powerful man was entirely recognizable.

Almroth Wright considered the submissiveness of women so ingrained and so natural, that he gave it a political dimension. His pamphlet *The Unexpurgated Case Against Woman Suffrage* was published, to great controversy, in 1913. Females, he argued, were deficient not just in physical force but also in the matter of intellect, and practically every man could detect this element of unreason:

> Woman's mind attends in appraising a statement primarily to the mental images which it evokes, and only secondarily – and sometimes not at all – to what is predicated in the statement. It is over-influenced by individual instances; arrives at conclusions on incomplete evidence; has a very imperfect sense of proportion.

She accepts the congenial as true, and rejects the uncongenial as false. In her private world, such an attitude might cause her to believe the false promises of a potential husband. In the political world, she is not equipped to assess matters of state.

Man, he thought, could assess a situation in unemotional terms – allowing him to be truly moral. The sinking of the *Titanic*, said Wright, showed 'in a conspicuous manner' that the ordinary man will sacrifice his own life to obey the communal law which requires him, when involved in a catastrophe, to save first the women and children. In this world, a woman would trust any man who said he had her interests at heart. He, after all, was her intellectual and moral superior – and her protector.

Almroth Wright went further. All women, he thought, should be married – for if they were denied their natural roles as wives and mothers, they were prone to turn political. 'The failure to recognise that man is the master, and why he is the master,' he wrote, 'lies at the root of the suffrage movement.' And, for her part, 'the happy wife and mother is never passionately concerned about the suffrage'. The best way forward for spinsters was emigration to countries such as Canada, where there was a shortage of women. (In fact, two years earlier, under the headline 'Searching for Five Thousand Wives', the newspapers carried reports of a Canadian immigration official who was touring the United Kingdom, 'holding meetings and making house visits' to find girls willing to become the wives of young Canadian farmers.) In Almroth Wright's terms, the compliant behaviour of George Smith's wives was understandable, and it was their misfortune that he was not a true man but an aberration.

It was also explainable from the feminist perspective of Cicely Hamilton. In 1909 she published her book *Marriage as a Trade*, arguing that girls, from a young age, are trained to be submissive, to please men. This, she states, is necessary because everyone knows they will be entirely dependent on marriage for their future livelihood. A man might be romantic, she says, but a woman cannot afford such a luxury. Instead, she must play a hard-headed game, appearing to be everything a man wants in the hope that he will pluck her from the poverty and disgrace that spinsterhood would bring. The *Strand Magazine* debate on 'What Sort of Woman a Man Likes' summed up the nature of her task in the contribution of Coulson Hernahan: 'She need not be clever, provided that she is clever enough to understand, to sympathise with and to idealise the man of her choice.'

In 1911 Hamilton published a novel *Just to Get Married* in which the heroine Georgina Vicary is in a dire situation: 'Either I go to a man who is willing or anxious to keep me, or I stay as a burden and a failure with the people who are longing to be rid of me' – the words might have been written by Margaret Lofty, living on slender means with her mother and sister. To secure a husband, says Cicely Hamilton, a woman should play a passive role – smiling, being gentle, womanly and admiring. There were, however, strict limits to her behaviour: she must never be forward, and in the end, it was up to *him* to choose *her*. In that respect, Coulson Hernahan was mistaken – a woman must idealize not the man of her choice *but the man who chooses her.*

In Eric Watson's view, if that man had made many sexual conquests he would be particularly attractive to women. George Smith, he says, was obviously such a man. 'It is a fact', he writes – expressing some puzzlement –

that a man has an easy task with women if he has the reputation of being a great hand with them. Perhaps this is only an expression of the conceit and envy of women, who cannot bear the idea that a man is interested in so many others and not in themselves . . . The inconceivable ease with which certain types of men seduce women, and at whose heads women throw themselves in spite of the fact that these men have no praiseworthy qualities whatever, can only be so explained.

As Samuel Johnson had noticed: 'the greatest profligate will be as well received as the man of greatest virtue, and this by a woman who says her prayers three times a day'. Although George's sexual swagger and self-regard was seen as misplaced and arrogant by many who met him, the argument ran, it may have seemed attractive to young women whose suppressed sensuality clouded their vision.

Watson's thoughts do not stretch to consideration of the miserable plight – economic, social and psychological – of the 'surplus woman', or to her sense of relief and deliverance when a man, almost any man, expressed a desire to marry her. Wives were proper women, a force for love in the family, and filled with womanly purpose. They had nurturing duties that filled the day: keeping the house, cooking the meals, etc. And, supported by their spouses' income, they could peruse the magazines and the clothes shops for feminine purchases: pretty dresses and fashionable hats. It seemed that wives had everything companionable and good, while single women were bereft and isolated in a harsher, colder world.

In this context George Smith had only to hint at a married future for the scent of orange blossom to put all other considerations in the shade. Doubts could be dismissed; his bullying behaviour interpreted as masculine and masterful. And his plans for the future might have seemed exciting. He said he was ambitious, and planned to set up an antiques shop. He wanted to travel – and endlessly referred to the promise of a trip to Canada.

For an ordinary girl, in an ordinary life, the negative might be suppressed in favour of the spark that came from George's unconventional nature.

Somehow this interpretation has most resonance in the cases of Bessie and Margaret, who gave the impression of being oppressed by their circumstances. Bessie seemed vulnerable because of her simplicity and passivity (she 'was always a woman who would be easily led', said her brother Howard), and Margaret because of her quiet, introverted character and her poverty. But Alice was different. She had a sunny, positive outlook, a good job and the support of an exceptionally strong family. Her susceptibility seems to have come from somewhere else. Quite probably the clue lies in the operation for septic peritonitis that she had just before she met George. This, it seems, was necessary because she was infected with gonorrhoea. 'Mr George Smith is aware of all that occurred' during this 'unfortunate incident' in Alice's life, wrote her doctor Bertram Stone.

In the days before penicillin, 'the clap' was all but untreatable. Women were given douches, and caustic substances were applied to the cervix – but many continued to suffer with painful urination and pelvic inflammatory disease, a complication which, without the sort of surgery that Alice had, could be fatal. Gonorrhoea could also make a woman infertile and was so common that it was considered a 'terrible peril to our Imperial race'. In 1909 a medical officer at the Liverpool Stanley Hospital estimated that one in seven of women out-patients, and a quarter of in-patients had gonorrhoea, and in 1913 the suffragist Christabel Pankhurst published her famous tract *The Great Scourge and How to End It*, in which she stated that gonorrhoea was 'the great curse of women and the cause of most of the special ailments from which they suffer'. Gonorrhoea was very easily caught, and poor Alice needed to have slept just once with a man to have picked it up. There can be little doubt that George would have maximized his use of the information, and threatened to shame Alice to her friends and family.

If the submissive behaviour of Bessie, Alice and Margaret was explicable, George's evil character was harder to interpret. In 1916 Sigmund Freud acknowledged that, in the course of his psychoanalytical work, he had come across 'those who commit crimes without any sense of guilt'. But there was not, as yet, any widely recognized concept of the psychopath. The first major work on the subject was Dr Hervey Cleckley's *The Mask of Sanity*, published in 1941. In the 1960s Robert Hare published a checklist of features associated with psychopathy which remains influential. Almost all of them apply to George Smith. The psychopath, says Hare, is prone to 'aggressive narcissism' – the chief features of which are glibness and superficial charm, a grandiose sense of self-worth, pathological lying, a cunning, manipulative nature, a lack of remorse or guilt and lack of empathy, and a failure to accept responsibility for his own actions. The lifestyle of the psychopath is determined by a need for stimulation, parasitic behaviour, poor behavioural control, promiscuous sexual behaviour, lack of realistic long-term goals, impulsivity and juvenile delinquency. In addition, the psychopath is prone to 'criminal versatility' and 'many short-term marital relationships'.

But this wasn't the language of 1915. Then George Smith's power seemed mysterious, explained less by a medical approach and more by the workings of the devil. His strange, evil power over women was made even more fascinating by the fact that women, in droves, turned up to see him each time he appeared at the police court. One paper, the *Weekly Dispatch*, started a campaign against the 'Women who gloat over the Brides' Case'. At Bow Street, said the paper,

women came journeys of fifty and sixty miles to catch a glimpse of him . . . they stood outside in a queue as early as eight o'clock in the morning in order not to miss the chance of a seat in court; they were content to sit sweltering amid a press of people the whole of a sunny day listening to the most tedious formal evidence in order that from time to time they could have a look at Smith in the dock.

It was part of George's mystique that he had used the language of love and romance to such devastating effect. Letters that he had sent to Caroline Thornhill were published as evidence of his 'honeyed tongue'. George, wrote the commentators, 'was full of soft honeyed phrases which he got from books. He adapted lines from Shakespeare and passed them off as his own. He borrowed gushing sentences from penny novelettes and made the women to whom he wrote think he was a man of passionate ardour'. His 'love vocabulary' to Caroline, commented the *Weekly Dispatch*, could be gauged from a selection of the endearing terms he used:

> You remain still my heart and soul.
> Your most loving husband.
> You are still my wife whatever happens.
> We cannot fully enjoy ourselves or anything else unless the
> one we love shares it with us.
> Heaven bless you, Caroline.
> Why did the very eyes of you make me so foolish, charm the
> very life of me, and make me a mad, loving fool?

For Arthur Neil the character of George Smith was of less concern than the amassing of evidence against him. During the spring of 1915 he and his officers set off on trips around the country, taking statements from relatives, landladies in seaside towns, lawyers who drew up wills, insurance agents who had insured lives and bank managers who had paid out money to George. It was reputed to be Scotland Yard's most extensive investigation ever. Neil collected 253 exhibits that could be used in court. They included marriage certificates, death certificates; letters, postcards and telegrams from George, plans of the houses in which the deaths occurred, Margaret's holdall containing her clothing, photographs of Bessie and Alice, the brass plate from the door of 80 High Street, Herne Bay, an umbrella, a Gladstone bag and three baths. At last, George Smith was charged with the murders of Bessie Mundy, Alice Burnham and Margaret Lofty – and it was then decided that he would face trial for the murder of Bessie.

George's solicitor, Walter Davies, decided to approach the country's top defence barrister – Edward Marshall Hall. The Great Defender had claimed that he would have saved Dr Crippen from the gallows; he had secured the freedom of Edward Lawrence when, to all the world, it had initially seemed that Lawrence had murdered his lover Ruth Hadley; he had tied William Willcox up in knots at the trial of the poisoner Frederick Seddon, and he had dismissed with a flourish the forensic evidence of Bernard Spilsbury at the trial of Jeannie Baxter, the woman who shot at Julian Hall four times, hitting him twice. His great theatrical summing-up speech had ignored the scientists, and persuaded the jury to believe instead a narrative of his own devising, put forward with such conviction that the fortunate Jeannie got away with a charge of manslaughter. Persuading a jury that Bessie Mundy had – as her doctor had testified, and an inquest jury believed – died accidentally in a bath following an epileptic fit, might have seemed, in comparison, an easy task.

At the outbreak of war Marshall Hall, now in his mid-fifties, was 'physically quite unfit for any form of active service'. So, he had to stay at home and in the words of the national war slogan, carry on with 'business as usual'. After the tragic early death of his first wife, Ethel, he had married a German woman, Hetty Kroeger, which was a difficult situation, given the public hatred of Germans. 'To Marshall Hall', wrote his friend Edward Marjoribanks, 'the most patriotic, sensitive and affectionate of men, the position was distressing in the extreme. He tended to see less of his friends and absorb himself even more than ever in his professional duties.'

Marshall Hall accepted the brief. But he was concerned that George had no funds with which to finance his defence. The police had taken possession of the £70 which he had in cash and were reluctant to hand it over. All the proceeds of the insurance policies on his wives' lives, and from their wills, were tied up in annuities – and George was now penniless. He had not even paid for the clothes that he had worn to his numerous police court appearances. So, when the press offered to pay his legal fees, in return for his life story – to be published after the trial – it seemed to Marshall Hall a good solution. But the Home Office refused to let George sign the contract. Marshall Hall objected. A man might sell his property to finance his defence. So why not his story, if that were his only asset? The row was still going on when the trial opened at the Old Bailey on 22 June.

9

Trial

O N THE NIGHT of 31 May 1915 the Zeppelins came to London. Thirty-five bombs and ninety incendiaries were thrown out of an airship, hitting residential streets in the East End. The first enemy bomb ever to fall on London from the air struck 16 Alkham Road, Stoke Newington. Others hit the narrow alleyways and streets of Whitechapel, Shoreditch and Hoxton. In Balls Pond Road, husband and wife, Henry and Caroline Good were, according to the *Daily Mirror*, kneeling in prayer by their bed when the bomb that fell on their house killed them. In death, Henry's arm was still round the waist of his wife. Her hand was full of her own hair, and the doctor at the inquest said he thought she had pulled it out in pain. Nearby, 3-year-old Elsie Leggett was sleeping in a room with her four brothers and sisters when a German bomb set their house alight. Her father managed to save her siblings, and was in hospital with severe burns, but Elsie died. In all, seven people, four of them children, died in the raid.

The deaths were, in number, tiny and insignificant compared with the tens of thousands of soldiers who were being slaughtered at the Front. But they caused a particular sort of outrage. These were 'innocent civilians', like the 1,198 passengers of the Cunard liner *Lusitania* who died in the Atlantic Ocean when the ship was torpedoed by a German submarine earlier that month. An attack on the wives, mothers, fathers, sweethearts and children of soldiers seemed the ultimate abuse. The German objective, it was commonly believed, was to demoralize the British people so completely that they would demand that their government surrender, and bring an end to the war. 'The Zeppelin has been built with the idea of spreading panic over as wide an inhabitant area as possible,' reported the *Evening Standard*. 'It has been devised as the terror of the air, the very quintessence of frightfulness.' The Germans, reported the *Weekly Dispatch*, measured their success with the Zeppelins, 'not by the few women or babies that are killed but by the degree of fear they hope to inspire'. And, in one respect, they were successful. The Zeppelin was, more than ever, a symbol of German technological superiority, a leviathan of the skies: unstoppable, unassailable. None of the nine British planes that went up to attack the airship over London that May had any effect, and one crashed, killing the pilot.

After the raids, the *Daily Express* drove home the symbolism by publishing a mocked-up picture entitled 'What a Zeppelin Raider Looks Like', showing the airship, 520 feet in length, hovering ominously over London's National Gallery – the ship being longer than the building. And the invincibility of the Zeppelin stoked the imaginations of those in the highest echelons of the armed forces. In a memorandum, Lord Fisher, the First Sea Lord, pictured, 'a Zeppelin holocaust from a ton of explosives dropped from the clouds on to Horse Guards Parade', which would, in one shattering explosion, kill all the Admirals, Generals, Statesmen and Civil Servants who were running the war.

The bombing raid was a propaganda victory for Germany. The Kaiser who, contrary to reports in the British press, had been reluctant to bomb London, now declared Count Zeppelin 'the greatest German of the twentieth century'. The response of the newspapers was to portray the Kaiser and 'Count Zepp' as the orchestrators of a policy of 'frightfulness and infanticide'. And the consequent public outrage produced anti-German riots across London.

The censored British press reported that Germans were convinced that their Zeppelins had caused 'mass hysteria' and 'moral insanity' amongst 'the whole of the English people'. In reality, though many Londoners were frightened by the Zeppelins, they were angry too, and refused to be cowed. The constant message 'business as usual' was relayed with new enthusiasm. To carry on as normal was the best tribute that London could pay to its sons who were fighting across the Channel.

The *Weekly Dispatch* told its readers that, far from causing hysteria, the Zeppelin attack 'has resulted in the emergence of a great national spirit of earnestness and self-sacrifice', though the paper thought the war might produce an increase in female insanity. 'Millions of the choicest and best of the young men in Europe will be killed off', and women will suffer

> the loss of husbands at the front and the dearth of potential husbands for the unmarried. It is an old but nevertheless true saying that men must work and women must weep . . . We all of us know heartbroken mothers whose only sons have been killed, while the strain on multitudes of women who are in constant suspense in regard to the fate of their loved ones is often quite as great.

Evil was turning the world upside down. There was the horror experienced by the men and boys at Mons, on the Marne and at Ypres, the terrible anxiety of their loved ones at home; and now the monsters of the sky attacking the nation's capital. The least that Londoners could do was to hold their nerve. Fortitude was demanded, and was forthcoming. In the days after the Zeppelin raid on London the calls for men to sign up and fight were made with renewed vigour. The *Daily Express*, one voice amongst many, proclaimed that '300,000 men are wanted at once . . . Unless you are making munitions, *your* duty is to Join the Army To-day.'

★

In the midst of the turmoil, a news story pushed the First World War off the front page. The opening of the trial for murder of George Joseph Smith was a sensation – reported in the newspapers of New York, as well as all the British papers. Wives and boarding-houses and baths were, for now, the riveting subjects of conversation. This homespun story was a diversion from the Zeppelins and the terrifying events in Europe, and it had a reassuring element to it. Here was evil that could be recognized and contained within the embrace of British justice – unlike the evil of war, which was rampant and beyond control. The characters in the story were familiar and drawn from a more innocent time. There was something girl-next-door about Bessie, Alice and Margaret – all of them nice, respectable young women. They were not the serious sort to go joining the suffragettes, nor the silly types – like Jeannie Baxter – who dolled themselves up in fashions and furs. They did not – like Cora Crippen – give themselves airs and graces. And were not – like Mrs Nowill – racy, modern women who played golf and went on Mediterranean cruises. They were the quiet, unassuming daughters of a bank manager, a fruit-grower and a clergyman.

It was public knowledge that more than a hundred witnesses were ready to testify against George Smith, the beast who, everyone believed, had betrayed his wives so cruelly. A hundred good people had cooperated with the police – relatives, doctors, undertakers, neighbours and, of course, landladies. And, leading the massive cast, were the lawyers who were to perform at the trial. The characters of Sir Archibald Bodkin, the barrister for the Crown, and Edward Marshall Hall for the defence were famous, since big murder trials, in a time before television, were national dramas and criminal barristers were celebrities. In addition, the plucky, resourceful policeman Arthur Neil was to testify. And, making his press début as the lead pathologist for the Home Office was Bernard Spilsbury – the young man who had so impressed at the trial of Dr Crippen five years earlier.

In the week before the trial, the papers published their curtain-raisers. The *Weekly Dispatch* seized the opportunity to continue its campaign against women spectators. 'Interest in the case has reached such an acute stage that there will be men as well as women to fight for the few seats available', it wrote, adding that 'if the women obtain half the seats they will have done well.' The paper pretended to be dismayed 'that any woman should be admitted at all to a trial that is bound to contain much medical evidence of a kind not suitable for everybody's ears'. And, the following issue was filled with a spirited condemnation of the voyeuristic types who attended the trial:

> As you pass the Old Bailey these June mornings that break either sullen and gloomy or are a flood of sunshine, you see a great crowd of well-dressed people surging up against the doors. The next day and the day after . . . still that same crowd. You wonder, when there is so much work to be done in England, why there should be this contemptible spectacle of an idling, lolling, gossiping, chattering assembly scrambling for admittance into a criminal court of the City of London as they might scramble for seats in a theatre, and as you wonder they whisper to you that inside a man . . . is being tried for murder.

As the doors were opened, the crowd surged forward, but only about a hundred people were admitted – the rest were left milling about on the pavement, waiting for news. Some of those who managed to gain entry did so not by joining the mob in the street but through their connections. A number of well-known people attended, amongst them, H. B. Irving – son of the great Victorian actor Henry Irving; George Sim, the novelist (and member of the Murder Club, to which Edward Marshall Hall, Arthur Conan Doyle and Bernard Spilsbury all, at various times, belonged); and the prolific writer of detective stories Edgar Wallace, who wrote an account of the trial for the magazine *Titbits*. He described the court 'packed tight with spectators, a large proportion of whom are women' and the reporters' desks which were 'crowded to their utmost capacity'. When George Smith makes his appearance, he writes, he comes up 'from the semi-darkness of the cells below to the strong light of day, and his eyes are narrowed as one to whom light is painful'.

> I have seen many men at the Old Bailey, guilty and innocent alike. I have seen murderers who were frankly bored by the proceedings. I have seen others who endured the anguish of death a hundred times a day. I have seen brute-men who were for all the world like wild beasts, and others, like Crippen, who have blinked at the Court in pained surprise that one so meek as they should find themselves in a position so much at variance with their conceptions of respectability.
>
> But such a man as George Joseph Smith I have not seen before.
>
> . . . The face is what the French call '*profond*'. The forehead is high and the well-brushed hair of dark brown, powdered at the temples with grey. He has a luxuriant moustache, and is obviously a man who takes a pride in his appearance. The lips are thin, the mouth straight and rather cruel, the jaw firm and obstinate, the nose straight and a thought 'pinched'. His eyes are curious. I had the feeling that I had seen them before, and remembered that I was comparing them with the eyes of a golden eagle.

When George told the court, at the outset of the trial, that he was 'not guilty', he did so in a clear, confident voice. Then he sat calmly, hands folded on his lap, paying attention as the proceedings began.

The prosecution barrister, Archie Bodkin, was 'tall and lean', the possessor of 'a magnificent physique', and a considerable athlete in his youth.

In terms of his height and bearing, he was a match for George's barrister, Edward Marshall Hall. But his approach was entirely different. He had no time for Marshall Hall's old-style theatrical mannerisms. Instead, his strength lay in his simple and direct manner, his attention to detail and mastery of points of law. His opening speech took seven hours – the entire first day of the trial – and was subsequently recognized as the best one he ever made. Mr Bodkin, 'suave-voiced, calm, official-mannered', began with George Smith's early life and his marriages first to Caroline Thornhill and then turned to Edith Pegler, who now became famous as 'the woman to whom he always returned'.

Bodkin described George's peripatetic existence, his long absences from Edith, and his sudden returns which were accompanied by an improvement in his finances. He then told 'the story of Miss Mundy' and George's keen interest in her money. When he came to the terrible letter that George had left for Bessie when he left her in Weymouth, accusing her of infecting him with a sexually transmitted disease, Bodkin said he would not read all of it – 'because there are things in it which I think I am absolutely justified in omitting. Let me tell you this, that these things which are omitted involve the grossest insults a man, let alone a husband, could offer to a woman who believed him to be her husband.' He wished to edit the letter to spare the blushes of the women in the public gallery.

But the judge, Mr Justice Scrutton, took a different view. 'No, Mr Bodkin,' he said. 'You must read the whole of the letter; if people come to Court to hear a case of this kind, they must put up with what they hear.'

His ruling delighted the *Weekly Dispatch*, which took another swipe at the 'motley collection of females' at the trial. 'They are very brazen women to sit there the whole afternoon listening to the sordid evidence that supports the case for the Crown.' But it infuriated campaigners for women's rights. Nina Boyle, the head of the political and militant department of the Women's Freedom League, fired off a letter to the judge. 'None of the women present had appealed to Mr Bodkin to spare them unpleasant details,' she wrote. 'And therefore his suggestion was purely impertinent and officious. If rebuke were called for, it was Mr

Bodkin who deserved it, for daring to suggest that the course of justice and the conduct of a Crown case should be altered because of the presence of the public in the enjoyment of its rights . . .'

The debate over the sexist conduct of the law, though, was a sideshow. The main focus was the effectiveness of Mr Bodkin's speech. 'You will notice,' he told the jury, 'there is not a thing in that letter which is not repeated three times over, and minute directions are given as to what she is to do, the part she is to play – just as if you were instructing a child – over and over again – nothing left to her, all set out in black and white, and repeated over and over again.'

He told the story of George and Bessie's life in Herne Bay, leading up to the day on which she, supposedly, had an epileptic fit and died in the bath. The fit, he contended, never happened. And the plausibility of the accidental death of a tall woman in a small bath was at issue. The inquest had been sloppy, he implied. And he made it plain that a post-mortem should have been held.

At this point, the jury withdrew. Mr Bodkin wished to persuade the judge to admit evidence relating to the deaths of Alice Burnham and Margaret Lofty. It is a principle of English law that evidence of the other crimes of an accused person is not generally admissible in court – and Edward Marshall Hall now vigorously opposed Bodkin's request. It was his firm view that if the evidence were confined to the circumstances of Bessie's death, he would save his client from the hangman. There was, after all, so much reasonable doubt in her case that the inquest jury had been convinced that her death was accidental. And the doctor in the case, Dr French, had not even thought it necessary to conduct a post-mortem. For him, clearly, there was no element of suspicion at all.

But Archie Bodkin was as determined to bring in the other cases as Marshall Hall was desperate to exclude them. And, faced with Bodkin – who was so adept at matters of law – and Marshall

Hall – who was known to struggle – and, of course, faced with the facts the judge, Thomas Scrutton, came down on the side of the Crown. The evidence relating to the deaths of Alice and Margaret would, he said, be admissible on the grounds that it related to the prosecution's intention to show 'system' – that the similarities between the cases was, in itself, evidence against George Smith. Marshall Hall argued that there was no prima-facie case relating to Bessie; so evidence of 'system' should not, in law, be allowed. But Scrutton disagreed.

Edward Marshall Hall's task became at a stroke vastly more difficult, and when the jury returned to court, Archie Bodkin 'quietly and with that easy flow of language which is his' went carefully through the stories of Alice and Margaret. George, wrote Edgar Wallace, 'follows Mr Bodkin's opening speech with the same keenness that a truculent shareholder might follow the recital of a company chairman's annual report. There is no sign of apprehension, none of fear, little of anxiety.'

George's physical presence in the courtroom was, for many, the most absorbing aspect of the trial. Here, within spitting dis-tance of the women spectators, a few feet away from grieving relatives, was the man himself – a distorted vision of masculinity that conjured up powerful images. While the young men of Britain were making the ultimate sacrifice for the sake of the nation, this man – strong and pugnacious - was the epitome of selfishness. He had no consideration for anyone around him, let alone a sense of duty to the nation. His drive and vitality, the Crown argued, had served only one purpose, to allay his sense of personal grievance. He exuded a sense of male forcefulness, and this was his overriding quality.

It gave him a power that some women found attractive, as H. B. Irving realized when he overheard two society ladies in the public gallery discussing the prisoner's magnetic appeal. A sense of sexual domination was in the air, and pervaded the atmos-phere as a procession of witnesses took the stand to give evidence about 'Henry's' relationship with Bessie, and a tale unfolded of his total domination of his wife. He treated her, it seemed, as though she had no will of her own, making all her decisions for her, being utterly cruel whenever it suited him. His high-handed, controlling manner was obvious when they were in the presence of other people, so how much worse might it have been when they were alone?

Bessie's Uncle Herbert appeared, and at once the sadness of her life was apparent. Even before she met 'Henry Williams', Uncle Herbert confirmed, she had drifted away from the family. After her father's death, her uncle never saw her again. 'She went to friends and to boarding-houses, or something of that sort,' he said. Her brother Howard said that he had seen her only 'from time to time'. Both men had known of the circumstances of her marriage only from her letters and the strange, malevolent, money-grabbing letters from Henry. There were no friends of Bessie to describe the circumstances of her romance, no intimates to whom she confided. Instead, the Weymouth landlady Maud Crabb and her husband Frederick were the closest people to her at the time of her wedding – and they both gave evidence.

Henry Williams had, said Frederick, claimed to have been a gymnasium instructor in the army. 'He asked me to feel the muscles of his arms, which I did, and found them to be very large.' George's pride in being physically strong on his wedding night was, of course, suggestive of sex, and once again conjured up a picture of the subjugation of Bessie. It was likely that she had never had sex before she met Henry, since respectable young women were expected to 'save themselves' for marriage. And now, submissive, passive and trusting, she was to experience love-making as this brute understood it. Who knows what happened behind closed doors in Weymouth and Herne Bay, but the very idea of sexual intimacy between Bessie and her husband was hard to take, as was the image of a young woman at her most vulnerable, naked in the bathroom, following her husband's command to keep the door unlocked so that he might enter. Bessie's last moments would, inevitably, be imagined in the context of sex, of subjugation and betrayal – and were particularly sad in the light of the testimony of Carrie Rapley, the Herne Bay secretary who rented out 80 High Street, and who now described Henry sobbing in her office after Bessie's death before adding, coolly and without emotion: 'Wasn't it a jolly good job I got her to make out her will?'

Solicitors took the stand, as did Adolphus Hill who had sold Henry and Bessie the 'five-foot bath with a plug in the bottom' and had taken it back a few days later. The bath, he said, was never paid for. Alfred Hogbin, the undertaker, appeared and told the court that Bessie had been buried in an unmarked grave. He had, he said, been present when her body had been disinterred. The next-door neighbour, Percy Millgate, gave evidence.

'I used to see Mrs Williams when I delivered bread to the house', he said. 'She came to the door nearly every day. She always seemed to be in good health when I saw her.'

'What sort of looking woman was she?' asked Archie Bodkin.

'Oh, very nice,' Percy replied, 'a dark-looking woman. She was a tall, medium-sized lady. The last time I saw her alive was on Friday morning, the 12th, when I was delivering bread. She was in perfectly good health that morning.'

The evidence of Dr Frank French reminded the jury, once more, of Henry's overbearing character. The doctor described the visit to his surgery, in which Henry spoke on Bessie's behalf, explaining that she had had a fit. He admitted that he had asked 'leading questions' of Mr Williams, raising the possibility of movements of the limbs and jaws. Henry had replied 'that the limbs were twitching and the jaws moved, that she opened and shut her mouth.' Dr French acknowledged, also, that 'she told me she did not remember anything about a fit, and that all she complained of the previous day was a headache.' Nobody questioned the doctor about his willingness to believe the husband

and not the wife. Nobody expressed the opinion that it was odd that she was not deemed capable of going to the doctor's surgery by herself – or of describing her own symptoms. The fact that her husband was treating her like a small child or an imbecile was not commented upon.

The doctor described visiting Bessie at home after her supposed second fit, when he found her 'sitting up in bed . . . She was flushed and had rather clammy, moist hands. The best way I can describe her condition is that she was as some one who had been recently wakened from sleep on a hot night.' Later that day he had seen Bessie again and she 'seemed to be in perfect health' but said she felt rather run-down. He described the morning of her death, how he had rushed to the house and found her lying in the bath, her head below the water-line.

At this point, the Herne Bay bath was brought into the courtroom. The judge asked Dr French to stand by the side of the bath, so that he could point to it when asked about Bessie's position, and could mark the water-line with a pencil.

'Her face was upward and partially submerged,' said Dr French, 'the mouth was in the water and, I think, the nostrils. Her legs were stretched straight out from the trunk. The toes of the feet were out of the water, resting on the end of the bath.'

The foreman of the jury then interjected. 'My lord,' he said, 'one of the jury has expressed a wish that some one should be put in the bath for ocular demonstration.'

The judge, though, did not wish events in the courtroom to take a farcical turn. 'I can only suggest to you,' he said, 'that when you examine these baths in your private room you should put one of yourselves in. Get some one of you to try it, who is about the height of 5 feet 9.'

Mr Bodkin returned to his examination of Dr French. When he had reached Bessie, said the doctor, he straight away felt her pulse – and there was none. He described his effort to revive her with artificial respiration. But Bessie, he said, was dead. Her face was bluish all over, and her body was entirely limp – except for the fact that in her right hand she clasped a square piece of Castille soap.

Edward Marshall Hall rose for the cross-examination and reminded Dr French that at the inquest into Bessie's death he had stated that there was nothing suspicious about it. Back then, he had been of the firm opinion that she had, indeed, died following an epileptic fit.

'Did you not say this before the coroner?' he asked: 'Her face was rather blue, as if she had met her death in an early stage of epilepsy. No signs of a struggle of any sort or shape, and in her hand a large piece of soap?'

'Yes,' replied Dr French.

'And that was your honest opinion at that time?'

'It was.'

Marshall Hall turned to the prosecution's theory that Bessie had been suddenly pulled up by the legs.

'If anybody,' he said, 'were to catch hold of her foot at the lower end of the bath and the bath was full of water, as you saw it, she would have ample opportunity of putting her arms across the outside of the bath to prevent her going under?'

Dr French thought that, yes, she would have been able to grab at the bath and struggle.

'Anybody,' continued Marshall Hall, 'would naturally and normally be expected to clutch the top of the bath?'

'Yes,' acknowledged Dr French. Nonetheless, he thought, it might be quite possible to drown someone that way, if they were very much surprised and the legs were rapidly drawn away.

'Did you make any examination of the body externally?' asked Marshall Hall.

'Yes,' said Dr French, and 'there were no marks at all.'

So, no signs of a struggle. And he admitted there was nothing in her appearance inconsistent with her having suffered an epileptic fit.

The Crown lawyer, Archie Bodkin, rose to ask Dr French more about the soap in Bessie's hand.

'Suppose,' he said, 'a person died suddenly with something in her hand, would that be still retained after death?'

'Yes,' answered Frank French, 'if they were grasping a thing.'

The judge now asked, 'If she fainted would she hold on to it?'

'I should think not,' said the doctor. 'I do not know.'

A note was passed by the jury to the judge.

'Supposing,' he said, 'a lady had lost consciousness through some sort of fit, what effect would it have on the grip of the hand on the soap?'

Dr French thought that if she died during the early stages of an epileptic fit, she might retain a grip on the soap. The early stages produced rigidity, he said, and the later stages limpness. It was noted that when Bessie was found, her legs were rigid – out straight, with her feet pressed against the end of the bath. In all, Dr French's evidence left plenty of room for reasonable doubt.

The long parade of witnesses to follow included the coroner Rutley Mowll, Alice Minter, who had laid out Bessie's body for a payment of five shillings, and a neighbour, Frances Stone, who had let Henry Williams sleep at her house in the days after Bessie's death.

'He was always late when he came in at night,' she said, 'except on one occasion when he came in about eleven o'clock, and I gave him his candle. After . . . he came down again and said, "It is no use; if I went to bed I could not sleep, I must go out again."'

'Did you notice his condition when he said that?' asked Archie Bodkin.

'Yes,' the witness replied, 'he looked very hot and frightened. He went out and I do not know when he came back again . . .'

And the baker's wife, Ellen Millgate, also noticed a nervousness in Henry when he slept at her house: 'he said he could not sleep without a light.'

The remainder of the evidence relating to Bessie's death came from bank managers and bank clerks in Herne Bay, Tunbridge Wells, Bath, Bristol and Weston-super-Mare, and from several solicitors. Her husband's sudden windfalls were recorded, along with his buying and selling of houses, and movements around the south of England. By the end of the third day of the trial he had arrived in Portsmouth, and the fourth day opened with evidence relating to the death of Alice Burnham. 'Henry Williams' was now George Smith.

William Knowles of Lloyds Bank told the court that on 2 October 1913 George Joseph Smith opened an account, giving his address as Kimberley Road, Southsea. This was the month in which he met Alice and persuaded her to marry him. On 8 October he paid in almost £1,300 – plainly the proceeds of Bessie's death. The account, said Mr Knowles, was closed on 23 January 1914 – a few weeks after Alice died. Charles Pleasance, a Southsea insurance agent, appeared next, and said that George had purchased an annuity with £1,300 in October 1913. He had told Mr Pleasance that he expected to buy a further annuity of about £500 the following January. The impression was created of George as a man who was planning and scheming – who had a clear vision of what his future income would be. Edgar Wallace wrote of the prisoner in the dock: 'There is the same fierce, unfaltering gaze, the same passionless stare, and a coldness which speaks of deliberation and forethought.'

Alice's father, Charles Burnham, took the witness stand and told the story of George's disastrous visit to Aston Clinton, and his outrageous, threatening letters were produced as exhibits. Charles' wife Elizabeth said Alice 'was very well in health'. She 'was a very bright girl; she went out in the fresh air and took exercise, and seemed to enjoy her life'. She told of the way in which she and her son Norman had rushed to Blackpool on hearing of Alice's death, and had attended her funeral. Under cross-examination, she acknowledged that her daughter had 'at certain times' suffered from headaches – meaning that Alice got headaches at the time of her period. In a way, the appearance of Alice's brother Norman was the most moving. He simply told the court that he had gone back to Blackpool to be present when his sister's body was exhumed, and had identified it.

Alice's doctor, Bertram Stone, told the story of her operation. The underlying ailment was not revealed in court. Instead, Dr Stone wrote it down on a piece of paper which was passed to the jury. 'The affection for which I was treating her was a local affection,' he said. Otherwise, she was in good health. He had, he said, examined her heart on several occasions and found it to be 'quite sound'. More landladies took the stand. Annie Page, who had rented out the rooms at 80 Kimberley Road, Southsea, testified that there was a bath at the lodgings, but no one, including Alice, ever used it. Susanna Marsden, who let rooms in Adelaide Road, Blackpool, said that George Smith had rejected her accommodation because there was no bath. And Margaret Crossley gave a lengthy account of the Smiths' stay at 16 Regent Road. George and Alice had arrived there on 10 December 1913, she said. 'Before they went upstairs I heard Smith mumble to Mrs Smith, and I could not make out what it was, and then she said, "Oh yes, have you a bath?"' Alice's health, she added, seemed to be 'quite all right'. She told of the water that came through the kitchen ceiling while Alice was taking her bath, said that the bathroom door had had a perfectly good bolt which Alice, for some reason, had not used. She made it clear that she had been suspicious of George Smith – largely because of his 'callous' behaviour after Alice's death. When Alice's body was still in the house Mrs Crossley had said: 'Now, Smith, you cannot stop here tonight,' and he said, 'Why, I could sleep where she was,' and I said, 'I take care you do not.' He replied, 'When they are dead they are dead.' At this point George shouted out from the dock, 'This woman is a lunatic!'

After the funeral, said Margaret Crossley, 'he came to fetch his hold-all, and stayed for about ten minutes. I remember his leaving his address.' The card on which George Smith had written his Southsea address was then produced. On the back of it, the landlady had written: 'wife died in bath, I shall see him again one day'.

'I suggest to you', said Edward Marshall Hall, 'that you have a very strong feeling against Mr Smith?'

'Oh no,' Mrs Crossley replied.

'And that you are colouring your evidence?'

'No,' she said, 'I am not.'

'Did he ask you why you would not have him in the house that night?' continued Marshall Hall, 'and did you say, "Because I won't have a callous man like you in the house"?'

'Yes.'

'What do you think made you say he was a callous man?'

'Because he did not seem to worry at all, for one thing,' said Mrs Crossley.

'Was he not very upset?'

'There is a difference,' she replied, 'between being in trouble and upset. I did not like his manner, and he knew I did not.'

Marshall Hall pointed out that at the inquest Mrs Crossley had not mentioned the water coming through the kitchen ceiling, and had not shown it to the policeman who came to the scene.

'You knew,' he said, 'that the inquest was for the purpose of inquiring into the cause of this unfortunate woman's death?'

'Yes.'

'If you had had any suspicion of the husband being concerned in the death, would it not have been your duty to have told the coroner?'

'It would not have been my business to say anything,' she replied weakly.

On the fifth day of the trial Mrs Crossley's neighbour Sarah Haynes told of how, when she cleaned the bath after Alice's

death, she found a vast quantity of hair at both ends. The policeman Robert Valiant told of lifting Alice's head out of the water,
and holding her until the doctor arrived. 'Did you make any note
at all of the prisoner's manner?' asked Mr Bodkin. The defence
objected to the question. The judge dismissed the objection, but
warned the jury to 'bear in mind that a good many people who
have seen nothing, when they are told something, they see a lot.
There is a good deal of that in all this evidence. The jury will be
careful and give weight to it.' On resumption of his evidence,
Police Sergeant Valiant said that George 'appeared callous and in
no way disturbed'.

Dr George Billing took the stand, and described Alice and
George Smith's visit to his surgery on 13 December 1913.
George, he said, had done the talking, saying his wife complained of headaches. He had prescribed tablets for her headache,
and a stomach medicine because she was suffering from consti-
pation. The next time he had seen Alice was in the bath at
Regents Road. 'The Blackpool bath' was now brought into
court, so that Dr Billing could mark with pencil Alice's position
in it - the point on the bottom of the bath where her buttocks
were resting, and the line on the side of the bath where her
shoulders were. When he arrived on the scene, he said, Alice's
head was at the tap-end. She was partly sitting, with George
supporting her. He could not see where her legs were because
the water was so soapy. The water, he said, was quite hot, and
the bath was filled to within a half an inch of the top. Had her
head been under water, of course, the water would have been
very near to the top of the bath. Alice, he said, had been fat.
And when he examined her body, he found fat surrounding the
heart and most of the organs. There was some fatty degeneration of her heart, in that the fat was just starting to get in
between the muscles. He also found some thickening of the
mitral valve, which he put down to the rheumatic fever she
had suffered as a child. However, 'it was not from any affection

of the heart that she died . . . the cause of death was, in my opinion, drowning.'

Under cross-examination, Dr Billing was quizzed about his testimony at the inquest.

'Did you say,' he was asked, ' "I take it that the hot water would act upon the heart and cause her to have a fit or faint. It was the heart affection which caused her to be mazy while she was in the water"?'

Dr Billing admitted that, at the time, he had thought the hot water in the bath might cause anaemia of the brain, or that she might have fainted in the bath. Again, he described the way in which Alice had been positioned in the bath, and said that, in his view, had she fainted it would be quite impossible for her head to have gone under the water at the narrow end of the bath.

The judge intervened. 'Did it strike you at all odd,' he asked, 'to find the head at that end of the bath?'

'Yes,' answered Dr Billing, 'very odd.'

The usual procession of undertakers, solicitors and insurance agents followed. John Robbins of the North British and Mercantile insurance company testified that on 17 January 1914 the £506 due on the death of Alice Burnham was paid into the account of George Joseph Smith at Lloyds Bank in Cheltenham. The sum was just as George had foretold – around £500, at the time he had anticipated – January 1914 – and he was in a position to buy another annuity.

The landladies in the case of Margaret Lofty now made an appearance. Harriet Smith of Bath told of renting out rooms to John Lloyd and Margaret Lofty in the days before their wedding. Emma Heiss and Ada Lokker in Highgate described how John Lloyd had been angry when they refused to rent him rooms without a reference. Then Arthur Lewis, an Islington solicitor, testified that Margaret Lloyd had been a stranger to him when, on 18 December, she came into his office and asked to make her will.

Further evidence was taken on the shape and size of the three baths, and the efficacy of the locks on the bathrooms.

Arthur Neil appeared, and described the effort it took to fill the Herne Bay bath – given the small downstairs boiler and its slow tap. 'In order to fill the bath half-way up,' he said, 'it would have required just over twelve journeys with that bucket, and to fill it three parts up it would have required over twenty journeys.' This seemed to put in doubt George's assertion that Bessie had run a bath and drowned in it in the half-hour that he had been out of the house buying fish. Neil said of the Highgate bath that 'I have been into the kitchen at 14 Bismarck Road. I was able in it to quite clearly hear sounds from the bathroom above, such as the pouring and splashing of water, and the rubbing against the bath.' The day ended with Mr Justice Scrutton addressing the jury. 'Gentlemen,' he said, 'you will have to consider this. This is a second lady who was a stranger in the house who has a bath with the door unlocked.'

Throughout these testimonies, George seemed curiously confident that the case was going his way. Edgar Wallace wrote that he sat in the court

> with a nonchalance and ease which suggests that he has been a constant visitor all his life . . . He is perfectly at home, incurious, detached. He favours the jury with a critical stare . . . There is no sign of apprehension, none of fear, little of anxiety. He glows at moments with righteous indignation and shakes his head in dissent when some statement is made of which he does not approve . . . The growing triumph of his manner as witness after witness faced the cross-examination of his counsel, Mr Marshall Hall, indicated how bright was the hope and how confident the faith within him.

The sixth day of the trial opened with the poignant testimony of Margaret's sister, Ethel Lofty: 'She had quite good health, I did not notice anything the matter with her in December, except that she was brighter and seemed happier.'(Plainly, moments of happiness had not come very often to Margaret.) 'I last saw my sister on 15 December,' continued Ethel. 'She left home that day about half-past one, saying she was going out to tea. I had no idea that she was leaving home except to go out to tea. I had no idea that she was engaged to be married at that time. I did not know anything of a man named Lloyd.' Her other sister, Emily, said that on 4 February she had come to London to go to the mortuary at Friern Barnet, where she had identified Margaret's exhumed body.

The Highgate landlady, Louisa Blatch, told the court that John and Margaret Lloyd had come to her house in Bismarck Road on 17 December last, and after ascertaining that she had a bath, had taken a room. 'Later on in the evening,' she said, 'I remember seeing Mrs Lloyd putting her outdoor things on again. As they were going out she said: "He wants me to go out with him a little while".' This was the last evening of Margaret's life – the one that she had spent visiting the doctor. In the morning, John Lloyd told Miss Blatch about Margaret's illness. They left the house for a while, bought fish, returned, and Margaret had her bath.

Louisa Blatch told the court that while she was busy in the scullery and the kitchen she had heard the sound of splashing in the bathroom, then a noise that seemed to be of hands or arms on the side of the bath, followed by a sigh. The next thing she heard was the playing of the organ. Then, after a while, came the sound of the front door shutting, shortly followed by the doorbell, rung by John Lloyd as he returned with 'tomatoes for Mrs Lloyd's supper'. She then relayed the story of Margaret's death – of John Lloyd calling out for help, of him telling her to send for Dr Bates, and asking whether he should let the water off. On the night of the death, she said, John Lloyd stayed in her house, sleeping in the downstairs sitting-room, while the body of his wife was in the bedroom. Miss Blatch added that the state of an article of

Margaret's clothing suggested that she 'was either in, or had recently been in, a period'.

Under cross-examination by Edward Marshall Hall the same questions came up. Why had the landlady not given the same evidence at the inquest that she was now giving at the Old Bailey? Surely, went his implication, the inquest evidence was more immediate, and more dependable, than evidence now tainted by unreliable hindsight? At the inquest Louisa Blatch had said nothing of the splashing, which she now acknowledged was simply the sound of 'somebody having a bath'. 'I did not mention it to the coroner,' she said, 'because I attached no importance to it.' As for the sigh – she admitted it was merely the sort of sound 'a woman might make washing her head'.

Marshall Hall also obtained from Miss Blatch the acknowledgement that, on the night of Margaret's death, a mere ten or twelve minutes passed between the time that she had heard someone going up the stairs, towards the bathroom, and then the sound of the organ being played in the sitting-room on the ground floor. That was just twelve minutes at the outside in which John Lloyd might have drowned his wife.

Police constable Stanley Heath described how, on arrival at 14 Bismarck Road, he found John Lloyd trying to resuscitate Margaret by working her arms backwards and forwards. The policeman took over, 'applying the Schaffer method of artificial respiration to the stomach', until the doctor arrived ten or fifteen minutes later. 'My suspicions were not excited,' PC Heath admitted to Marshall Hall, 'there was no sign of any trouble or disorder.'

Dr Stephen Bates next related the story of the visit of John and Margaret Lloyd to his surgery, of her headache, her high temperature and her quick pulse. When cross-examined by Edward Marshall Hall, Dr Bates said that when Margaret had come to see him with her husband, 'she appeared to be dazed' and 'simply did not answer questions'.

'Did you find,' asked Marshall Hall, 'that she was, as far as you could judge, depressed?'

'She was,' answered Dr Bates.

'Did you say that you first feared mental trouble when you found the temperature high?'

'When I first saw her and found she would not answer questions, and stared vacantly about her, I did think so.'

Bessie and Alice had been quiet and passive at their pre-death visits to the doctor. Margaret was different. Of the three brides, she was the only one to be taken to the doctor actually on her wedding day – and maybe it was because of this that she was not just submissive but also stunned and bewildered. Perhaps it was dawning on her that she had made a horrendous mistake in marrying John. And, of the three women, she was the only one who was obviously genuinely ill – who was physically weak, as well as emotionally battered. The contrast with John Lloyd – healthy, sexual and predatory – was stark. 'His hands are heavy and strong,' wrote Wallace, 'and indeed sheer strength is his keynote.'

Dr French, on seeing the couple, concluded simply that the husband was healthy and the wife had influenza.

'Assume for the moment,' continued Marshall Hall, 'that she was suffering from the particular form of epidemic influenza at that time, complicated, as I suggest to you, by the presence of a period, would not the hot bath be the very worst thing she could possibly have?'

'Yes, I should say so.'

'. . . Assuming,' said Marshall Hall, 'a woman faints in a bath and is subsequently drowned without recovering consciousness, would the objective symptoms be those of fainting or death by drowning?'

Dr Bates replied, 'death by asphyxia [due to drowning]'.

'Therefore,' continued the counsel, 'from the objective symptoms it would be impossible to say the fainting fit had not preceded the drowning?'

'Exactly.'

The Highgate undertaker, Frederick Beckett, told of John Lloyd's insistence on a public grave for his wife, and his objectionable bargaining over the price of her funeral. And police sergeant Harold Reed took the stand to say that he had found a hold-all containing Margaret's clothing at John Lloyd's rented rooms in Shepherds Bush. He had also found there a list written out by 'Lloyd'. The words were mundane enough, but their significance was chilling: 'certificate of birth, certificate of marriage, certificate of death, wife's will, policy, receipt for premium paid, official acceptance, receipt for burial'. On the back of the paper was the receipt for a funeral, the number of an insurance policy – 26595 – and a date – 24.12.1914.

At this point, the judge asked the jury to retire so that he could hear a submission from the defence counsel. Edward Marshall Hall put up a spirited objection to the two prosecution witnesses who were to appear next – the lead Home Office pathologist on the case, Bernard Spilsbury, and the toxicologist William Willcox. Spilsbury and Willcox, Marshall Hall argued, could give evidence only on their area of expertise – that drowning was the cause of death. But the fact of drowning was not disputed by the defence. It was, said the barrister, entirely up to the jury to say, after hearing all the circumstances, *how* such drowning occurred. But Mr Justice Scrutton held that he could not exclude the expert evidence. So the jury returned, and Bernard Spilsbury took the stand.

10

Forensics

O N 28 JUNE the trial entered a new stage. 'Dr Spilbury's Evidence' was now the main focus. 'Did they Die During Fits?' asked the *Morning Advertiser.* 'Dr Spilsbury's Opinion'. The *Daily Express* added another dimension: 'Dr Spilsbury', it informed readers, is a clean-shaven, athletically-built, handsome man with jet black hair and alert, thoughtful eyes.'

On taking the stand, Spilsbury gave his credentials: 'I am a Bachelor of Medicine and a Bachelor of Surgery of Oxford. I am Pathologist at St Mary's Hospital. I have had a very extensive experience in not only making post-mortem examinations, but in dealing with a variety of conditions of the human body.' This last part was a neat glossing over of the fact that Spilsbury had very little experience of taking care of live patients – other than in examining samples taken from their body parts.

His account of his examination of Bessie's body emphasized 'the condition of the skin known as goose skin' that he found 'about the thighs and abdomen'. This phenomenon, he said, 'occurs in some cases of sudden death, and perhaps more frequently in sudden death from drowning. It is a sort of corrugating of the surface, a roughening of the surface.' The very fact of the goose skin, he was sure, indicated a very sudden death. Alice's body, he said, was in an even more advanced state of decomposition than Bessie's. He emphasized her size and the thickness of the fat over her breasts and buttocks. 'She was big bodied,' he said, 'from the shoulders and round the hips, and the hips were tightly wedged in the coffin.' Like Dr Billing, he noticed a slight thickening of the mitral valve in the heart.

'A person possessing a mitral valve with a slight thickening such as I found in this body would not be liable to sudden collapse,' he said.

'Do you think,' asked Archie Bodkin, 'that condition of the thickening of the mitral valve affected her health in any way?'

'No,' he replied, 'I do not.'

'Was there anything else wrong with her body at all that you could find?'

'No, nothing at all.'

In Margaret's case, Bernard Spilsbury noted that he had found traces of three bruises on her arm, rather than the one found at the first post-mortem. But he had 'found nothing to indicate any weakness or liability to faintness or collapse'.

He next demolished the idea that Bessie had had an epileptic fit. It would, he said, be unusual to have an epileptic fit for the first time over the age of 30. When a person had a fit, he said, they would most likely not be in normal health for the next day or two. And, if two fits occurred – as Bessie's husband had maintained – then the effect would be more pronounced still. And Bessie, according to witnesses, had seemed to be in good health after her supposed fits.

Then he turned to the baths. Noting the dimensions of the three baths, their narrowness at the bottom ends and the slopes at the base, he went through the various positions that someone might assume.

'If,' asked Mr Bodkin, 'the collapse had taken place kneeling facing the foot end might a person be drowned?'

'I think probably not,' said Spilsbury, 'because the kneeling position would have to be near the foot-end of the bath. They would not kneel in a very sloping part, and kneeling otherwise would bring the face over the taps or over the end of the bath.'

'Strike the head on the end of the bath?'

'Yes, or even strike the chest.'

'Strike the face on some part of the bath?'

'Yes.'

If a woman were sitting at the broad end of the bath looking towards the foot-end, Spilsbury thought, she 'might fall backwards rather than forwards and it is highly improbable, and I think in two of these baths, almost certainly impossible, if not quite so, for the head to become so submerged as to cause death by drowning.' He was, he said, speaking of the Blackpool bath and the Herne Bay bath.

And so Spilsbury continued – meticulously going through sitting, kneeling or standing in the bath, facing either end. If a woman were to fall face downwards while kneeling facing the sloping end of a bath, he thought she would drown. Similarly if she fell from a standing position facing that end. But in the most usual positions that a woman might assume in a bath, he calculated that she would not drown. If lying soaking, he observed, her head would rest on the end of the bath and would not be submerged.

'May I add to that,' said Spilsbury with great authority, 'usually a lady taking a bath of that sort would have the head completely out of the water; they do not usually wet their hair when taking a bath.'

Archie Bodkin asked Spilsbury to consider the position in which Bessie was found, with her head underwater, and her legs stretched out and raised, resting at the top of the bath.

'Can you,' he asked, 'give us any help at all as to how a woman could get into that position who has suffered an epileptic fit.'

'No – I cannot.' The pathologist was quite certain that if someone died during the first stage of epilepsy, when the body goes rigid, then their legs might be extended and stiff – but would not slope upwards as Bessie's had done. He was contemptuous of George's claim that he had raised his wife's head and rested it on the side of the bath, only to find her submerged, with her legs raised, when he reappeared with Dr French. Spilsbury said, categorically, he could give no scientific explanation for such a train of events.

In the case of Alice, taking into account her bulk and the narrowness of the bath, it was still possible for her to have drowned accidentally had she been kneeling or standing facing the sloping end. However, he said, it would be 'impossible' for her to have drowned as a result of a fit had she been sitting or lying in the bath. In the sitting position, with her back to the tap-end, and facing the foot-end, said Spilsbury, 'I think it would be impossible again for submersion of the face to occur.' It was noted that this was Alice's position in the bath when Dr Billing arrived at Regent Street and found Alice there, dead. The same observations, about sitting, standing, kneeling or lying, he asserted confidently, held true for Margaret.

As for fainting in a bath – it was most unlikely to cause death. Water, said Spilsbury, would pass into the windpipe, having 'a very powerful smarting effect, and would probably recover the person from the faint'. How long, asked Bodkin, might someone survive if they were submerged for a period of time, without being able to come up for air?

'If submersion were complete,' responded Spilsbury, 'the longest period during which the patient could survive would be about five minutes; and death would probably ensue in less than that time, and in some cases it might be either instantaneous or within a few seconds.'

'Do you mean', asked Bodkin, 'a case of sudden immersion?'

'Yes,' answered Spilsbury, 'in a case of sudden immersion, whether or not it was expected, consciousness would be lost at once . . . Immediately.'

A person who was submerged would be able to make 'muscular efforts', he continued, that is, to struggle and try to save themselves, unless unconsciousness came on very rapidly. The line of questioning supported the prosecution's theory that

George had pulled up his victims' legs, causing their heads to be submerged so suddenly that they passed out and died instantly.

Bodkin turned to the question of the soap in Bessie's hand. Spilsbury said that if the person were conscious when suddenly submerged, and a struggle ensued, she would grasp at any object within reach.

'Supposing the person having something in the hand suddenly loses consciousness from submersion,' said Bodkin, 'could you give us any opinion about that?'

'If only consciousness is lost,' replied Spilsbury, 'the soap or any other object would probably drop out of the hand by relaxation . . . But if death occurred immediately the contraction of the muscles of the hand might pass instantaneously into the death stiffening, and the object might be retained after death.'

'Supposing a person happening to have something in his hand fainted?'

'The fact of fainting,' said Spilsbury, 'would cause relaxation of the muscles and anything in the hand would be released.' In the first stage of an epileptic fit, 'anything which was grasped in the hand would probably be retained in the hand, but in the second stage, during the movements of the body, it is more likely that such an object would fall out of the hand again, and would certainly fall out in the third stage of exhaustion.' And if someone had some soap in their hand during a sudden death, he confirmed, it would be retained in the hand, 'owing to the condition of instantaneous death stiffening.'

Edward Marshall Hall now rose. 'Do I understand you to say,' he said, 'that you have come to the conclusion that in the Herne Bay case . . . accidental death was so improbable as to amount in your mind to impossibility?'

'Almost to impossibility,' Spilsbury replied.

'Almost — I will accept your candid admission; you say almost?'

'Yes.'

'The soap is a very difficult problem?'

'It is.'

'There is no theory under which you can deal with the clutching of that soap satisfactorily with the theory of a violent death – no absolute theory; you have got to make some qualification?'

'I think,' replied Spilsbury, 'one would assume a violent death in order to account for the soap being there.'

'. . . A violent death from an outside agency, that is to say from a person deliberately murdering her?'

'Yes.'

'The clutching of the soap does lend some probability to the theory of epilepsy?'

'It is not impossible; it is not very likely.'

'. . . Could you possibly force a piece of soap into a person's hand in simulation of its having been clutched in the act of death?'

'I do not think you could.'

Marshall Hall turned to the question of the impact of a cold, or coldish bath on someone who was hot and clammy after a very hot night.

'If a woman whose temperature has been raised by a night in bed like that, the bath having been prepared overnight, suddenly gets into a cold bath, there would be considerable shock?'

'There might be; it is partly a matter of surprise.'

'Anybody getting into a bath normally . . . would get in somewhere about the middle?'

'They would get in on the flat part on the bottom, certainly.'

'. . . In your experience have you had the misfortune of getting into a bath and as you were sitting down slipping up?'

'Yes I have.'

'In which case, of course, your feet would come down out of the water?'

'Well, not out of the water, they would come down to the bottom of the bath . . . The feet would certainly go forward, but I do not think they would go upwards.

'Would not they?'

'I do not think so.'

'. . . Is it your carefully formed opinion that this woman never had been subject to any form of epileptic fits?'

'None of the evidence I have heard seems to point to that, I think.'

'George Smith's statement was that he had raised the body and propped the head up on the side of the bath, and it might have slipped back,' said Marshall Hall. 'You do not think that would have happened?'

'I cannot account for that.'

'Is death by drowning in any sense of the word a very sudden death?'

'It depends upon whether the submersion is complete.'

Marshall Hall asked at what point 'death would supervene' after immersion in the water, assuming that Bessie had been drowned by George. Spilsbury answered 'immediately', within a matter of a second or two 'from the shock'.

Marshall Hall considered the theory of the pulling of the legs. Would it not, he asked, be very difficult to ensure that the victim's nostrils would go under the water, especially since the amount of water in Bessie's bath only reached about half way up the sides? But Spilsbury responded by observing that the body falling into the water would cause the water-line to rise, and the nostrils to go under. Surely, countered Marshall Hall, the assailant would need to push on the head to keep it under the water, and would not that produce tell-tale marks on the head? No, retorted Spilsbury, the pressure would definitely not produce marks. Marshall Hall changed tack. What, he asked, would a victim be doing with her hands at the moment in which she had her feet whisked up into the air?

'If she remains conscious,' said Spilsbury, 'she is making efforts clutching at anything that was near.' Thus, he brought the argument back to the soap.

Marshall Hall seemed incredulous. Do you really mean to say, he asked, that she would grasp the soap 'instead of putting up her hands to save herself from being pulled down?'

'Once under the water,' replied Spilsbury, 'she would be unable to do anything.'

But, said Marshall Hall, 'the moment she sees anybody – this man – clutching hold of her feet to pull them up she has only to drop the soap . . . and seize hold of each side of the bath' and he would be unable to submerge her.

'It is all a question of surprise,' said Spilsbury.. 'If it is done sufficiently quickly there would not be time to do that.'

But, said Marshall Hall, she cannot be surprised so much by a person who is in front of her, as she would be by someone attacking her from behind.

'She might not be alarmed by the approach,' said Spilsbury.

'But surely she would be alarmed by him reaching for her feet and lifting them up?'

'By the time that process is commenced, the whole thing would be done.'

'Would not the struggling be instinctive – almost automatic?'

'It would take a moment for the struggle to develop.'

Marshall Hall now turned to Alice's bath. Spilsbury would agree, would he not, that the temperature of her bath was quite high – about 104 degrees?

Spilsbury agreed.

'And that ladies, especially nurses, are very clean people?'

'Yes, they are.'

'. . . Have you known of women washing their heads in the bath?'

'They may wash their hair in the bath,' he now thought.

Marshall Hall suggested that Alice may have been kneeling in the bath, facing the taps, and bending under them to wring the soap out of her hair, when she fainted and drowned.

'I think,' responded Spilsbury, 'it would be almost impossible for her to rinse her hair in that bath in the position you suggest.'

'If the water will pour from the tap to the bath, it will equally pour over her head?' said Marshall Hall.

'It wants,' said Spilsbury, 'a certain amount of clearance.'

'. . . I agree,' said Marshall Hall, 'it involves getting her head down more than if there was a greater clearance between the tap and the bath?'

'Quite so.'

'The mere fact of bending the head down might cause a flow of blood to the head?'

Mr Justice Scrutton intervened. 'I do not follow this,' he said. 'What is supposed to happen – that she is in the water and putting her head under the tap?'

'She puts her head under the tap,' said Marshall Hall, 'turns the tap to get it running, and then faints.'

'And the water goes on running?' said the judge.

'And the water goes on running,' Marshall Hall agreed. 'Suppose the water goes on running, or supposing there is time for her to turn the water off, and she faints in the act of getting back, would it not be possible?'

'I do not think so,' said Spilsbury.

His imaginative scenario thus dismissed, and appearing somewhat desperate, Marshall Hall turned to Alice's state of health. Referring to the 'condition' – the unmentioned gonorrhoea – that led to her surgery, did it not 'leave its traces?' Does it not have 'a serious weakening effect?' Was it not 'a great drain on the system?'

'Yes,' answered Spilsbury to all these questions.

'It must be, must it not, that a woman who up to November has been receiving medical care on account of an illness of that kind would be more likely to have a fit than a woman in perfect health?' A fit, in December, that is.

'I do not think it would make any difference,' answered Spilsbury.

But the fatty degeneration of the heart would, Marshall Hall suggested, create a small disposition to faint?

'Yes.'

'In all faints, the difficulty is the failure of the heart to save the situation?'

'That is so, yes.'

The defence lawyer moved swiftly on to Margaret. She had had, he observed, a temperature of 101 degrees. Her doctor believed her to have been suffering from epidemic influenza, compounded by a gastric condition and 'nervous depression'. All this, he said, might be a serious factor in considering the case of sudden death in a hot bath.

'It is possible,' acknowledged Spilsbury, 'it would depend on the degree.'

And the bruises on Margaret's arm: 'how do you think they were caused?'

'I think in all probability, and assuming they actually occurred at the time of death, they were caused by blows against the side of the bath by the arm.'

But, said Marshall Hall, if bathing with a temperature of 101 degrees, Margaret 'had felt a sense of faintness and fallen down, would she naturally or very likely have bruised her arm?'

'She might have done so.'

So, said Marshall Hall, although you think it highly improbable that her death was due to an accident, 'you would not say absolutely impossible'?

'No,' acknowledged Spilsbury, 'not absolutely impossible.'

Archie Bodkin now asked whether, given the dimensions of the three women and the respective baths in which they were found, 'is the death of each of them consistent, in your judgement, with the suggestion . . . as to their legs having been lifted up and their heads submerged?'

'Yes.'

'And sudden death thereby resulting?'

'Yes.'

Bodkin returned to the clutching of the soap. Spilsbury had said that he had come across the phenomenon before – would he tell the court about that experience?

'The one which I have in my mind,' replied the doctor, 'is that of a man coming apparently unexpectedly into cold water – deep water – on a night carrying an electric torch in his hand; and when found some three weeks afterwards the electric torch was still firmly grasped in his hand.' In this case, the man's death was an accident. He appeared to have fallen into a reservoir.

As Spilsbury left the witness-box, he seemed like some fantastic scientific detective – having given such confident expert testimony on so many subjects – falling, bruising, bending, grasping, fainting, heart disease, epilepsy, shock, the hair-washing of women, and of course drowning. His colleague William Willcox was next to take the stand; his role being to support the evidence of the younger, more glamorous man. Willcox endorsed Spilsbury's view that it was highly unusual for a woman to have an epileptic fit for the first time at the age of 35. And he agreed that, if someone were submerged in water suddenly, without warning, they might become unconscious within a few seconds. 'In some cases,' he said, 'death may occur very quickly from shock.'

'That is death from drowning?' asked Mr Bodkin.

'No, it would be death from shock.'

'Might death from drowning, if a shock caused unconsciousness, rapidly supervene?'

'Yes.'

'. . . Is grasping of the soap in the hand consistent, in your opinion, with death from drowning in which sudden shock has occurred?'

'Yes,' replied Willcox, 'in death from drowning associated with shock or surprise; immediately after death, instantaneous death, stiffening is likely to occur; and hence the muscles holding the object remain contracted, and the object is held after death.'

'Just as to the evidence given by Dr Spilsbury?'

'Yes . . .'

'Supposing,' said Bodkin, 'that a woman were sitting in the ordinary position in a bath, and suddenly and unexpectedly her legs were raised, would her body tend to go along the body of the bath?'

'Yes, that would be so.'

'And in your judgement [given the amount of water that was said to be in the bath, and given the water displaced by the body] would there be sufficient water to submerge her head?'

'Yes, in my opinion there would be sufficient and two or three inches beyond that which would give it complete submersion.'

He continued on much the same lines, agreeing with Spilsbury's evidence about Alice's general good health, the effect of Margaret's temperature, and the implausibility of George's claim that he had left Bessie's head lying out of the bath, and returned to find her submerged, with her legs straight out. In fact, he said, he knew of no natural causes which could account for the position of her feet.

'May I take it you heard Dr Spilsbury's examination-in-chief?' continued Bodkin.

'Yes.'

'. . . May I take it if I put same or similar questions to you that your answers would be the same as Dr Spilsbury's?'

'Yes.'

Willcox's appearance brought the forensic evidence to its conclusion. The remainder of the prosecution's case was dominated by one more witness – Edith Pegler, 'the woman to whom he always returned'. She was dressed neatly 'in a blue costume', reported the *Daily Express*, 'and steadily faced counsel without once turning towards the man in the dock'. At last, the court and the press could properly inspect the modest, unassuming Edith. Could she really have had no idea that her husband was, at the very least, a serial bigamist and a conman? Did she suspect that he had the capacity for murder? Did she think that he had genuine feelings – like other people – of sympathy, love and compassion? As she began addressing the court, it was apparent through her straightforward, unembellished answers, that she had indeed been totally deceived by George. That she knew him to be a teller of tales, shifty and sly. But she had had no idea of his true nature.

She described her life with George – the constant moving about, the long absences and his intermittent income. 'I do not remember him mentioning any places where he had been', she said. She had known nothing of him marrying someone at Weymouth, or using the name of Williams. She remembered him being away for several months in 1913 – when he had met Alice – and told of him returning home saying 'he had just come from Spain. He told me he had bought some old-fashioned jewellery which would bring him about £200 eventually . . . I had no knowledge that the prisoner had been at either Portsmouth or Southsea, or that he had been married there. I also had no knowledge that he had been to Blackpool.'

When George went off to marry Margaret, he had told Edith he was going to London. He was away only ten days.

'I have no knowledge whatever,' said Edith, 'of his having been married to a Miss Lofty at Bath, or of his having assumed the name of Lloyd.'

'In taking apartments at various addresses you went to,' asked Bodkin, 'did you ever hear him ask if there was a bathroom?'

'At Weston-super-Mare he asked for one.'

'. . . Is that the only place you can recollect?'

'Yes. I think the prisoner had a bath there.'

She did not remember him having more than a few baths, ever.

During his cross-examination, Marshall Hall said: 'You know nothing, of course, of his having been mixed up with any other women at all? . . .'

'Nothing whatever,' replied Edith. She acknowledged that, before she knew anything of his bigamous marriages and the deaths of his wives, she had been fond of him.

'He had always treated you kindly?' asked the barrister.

'Yes.'

'In all the towns you went to I suppose there are public baths?' he continued.

'Yes.'

'And people in that position of life who have not got baths in their houses will have baths at the public baths?'

'I have heard that is the case.'

'You do not suggest that in all these six or seven years he had only one or two baths?'

'No; I should not think so.'

Finally, Arthur Neil re-entered the witness box to answer routine questions about the identification of the prisoner. The policeman's presence in the courtroom drove George into a rage. 'He suddenly rose from his seat', reported the *Daily Express*, 'his face white with passion, looked towards the judge and shouted – "You can't sentence me to death. I've done no murder!"' It was evident 'that he was in a state bordering on collapse. Tears fell down his pale cheeks. He tried to master them by closing his eyes. He covered his face with his left hand to hide his tears, but he finally gave up the struggle and for a full minute wept bitterly, with his handkerchief to his eyes.'

Archibald Bodkin's summing-up speech relied overwhelmingly on the forensic evidence given by Bernard Spilsbury, and corroborated by William Willcox. The gentlemen of the jury, he said, should start with the fact that George Smith is a systematic bigamist. His motive for the alleged crime is love of money, which is his 'predominant passion'. They should, he said, consider Bessie's supposed epilepsy. Spilsbury had said that epilepsy commencing at the age of 35 was 'most unusual'. Bessie 'had never had it before; she had no recollection of ever being unconscious. She was a healthy woman.' In fact, he said, it was extraordinary that for a 'mere headache' a person should think it necessary to go at once to see a doctor. 'The importance of that is that you find precisely the same condition of things repeated in the Blackpool and Highgate cases.'

Turning to the position of Bessie's body in the bath at Herne Bay, 'is it not clear', he asked, 'that a powerful man could pull up a woman's legs to move her body down in the water and submerge her face?'

> That involves the lifting of the legs, and the legs were found raised . . . you have it on the considered testimony of Dr Spilsbury and Dr Willcox that this death could easily have been caused in that way, and that it might have been, and that there was evidence that it was a sudden death. And if it were a sudden death, the whole of the circumstances are explained, down to the clutching of the piece of soap in the hand. A reason for saying that it was a sudden death is something which the doctor and the coroner's jury did not see, and that was the 'goose flesh' on the skin.

The medical evidence, he said, should be taken in conjunction with the circumstances. Who would benefit from Bessie's death? And was her death part of a system of deliberately causing deaths for monetary benefit? The three deaths, he continued, 'are of such a character that such a large aggregation of resemblances cannot have occurred without design' – and he listed the resemblances: the wills, the life insurance, the visits to the doctor, the letters to the relatives, the enquiries about baths, the deaths from drowning, the fact that George was first on the scene, the unfastening of the bathroom doors, 'and in each case the prisoner was putting demonstrably forward the purchase of either fish, or eggs, or tomatoes to show that he was absent from the house in which his wife was lying dead.'

Edward Marshall Hall had called no witnesses for the defence, and had decided against putting George Smith on the stand. This gave him the opportunity of speaking last, and he now led the oratory at the Old Bailey away from prosaic references to fish, eggs and tomatoes to the sombre image of the administration of justice while the world was at war.

> Gentlemen of the jury, this case is without parallel in the history of English crime, and very extraordinary from any point of view. At a moment like the present, when the flower of our youth are laying down their lives for their country, does it not strike you as a great tribute to the national character of level-headedness that, with all the panoply of pomp and law, we have been assembled day after day to inquire into the facts of this sordid case, and to decide whether or not one man should go to an ignominious death? . . . It is a great tribute to our national system of jurisprudence.

It was typical of his style to summon up the grandest of stages for his performance, and to seize the high ground whilst defending the most squalid of crimes.

He attacked the prosecution for the role it had given Bernard Spilsbury.

> The calling of expert medical evidence . . . has opened the door to the worst form of Americanism in the administration of British justice. Had the prisoner not been the pauper he is, had he been possessed of unlimited means like some recent American criminals, he might have procured experts to say that the cause of death was other than that stated by the experts for the Crown. I submit it is a very dangerous procedure that should be watched

with the greatest possible care and an absolute limit put on it. It has reached its extreme limit in this case.

His suggestion, of course, carried the implication that, had George been rich, an expert for the defence might have been found to argue that the goose skin was not definitive evidence of a sudden death, neither was the clutching of the soap. Or to discredit the 'sudden death' theory associated with the legs being pulled up. Or to say that the arrangement of falling bodies in baths was not taught at medical school. But all of this was unsaid. George had not been allowed to sell his story to finance his defence, an expert had not been sought, never mind found, and the forensic evidence, despite Marshall Hall's efforts, remained unchallenged in any substantial way.

Turning to the circumstantial evidence, Marshall Hall conceded that the prosecution had shown that George Smith had a motive for murder. However, the judge had said that 'motive may be an important factor, but it cannot convert suspicion into proof'. And, Marshall Hall continued, it should be remembered that the policies taken out on the lives of Alice and Margaret were 'endowment' and not 'all-life' – which would have delivered twice the benefits. If George were considering murdering his wives, and if he were so motivated by money, why did he not take out an all-life policy? And, if the prosecution was right in its conclusions, then 'the prisoner has committed one of the most diabolical of crimes that any records of any country have ever produced. One has to go back for a parallel to the days of the Borgias, when systematic poisoning extended over a period of years.' He urged the jury to think of the evidence of Edith Pegler. 'She admitted that he was always fond of her, and implied that she was fond of him, and that she had forgiven him that which women found the most difficult to forgive, his infidelity to her. Can this man be the unmitigated monster suggested by the evidence for the Crown?'

He now made a last-ditch attempt to undermine the evidence relating to the quick submersion of the women – evidence deemed to be within the area of expertise of Bernard Spilsbury. The theory put forward by the prosecution, he said, is that the prisoner murdered the woman by pulling up her feet, and so drowning her.

> I maintain that if you take the trouble to examine the bath and take the measurements of it and of the body, it is physically impossible to drown the woman in that way in eight inches of water; it is impossible and it is incredible . . . If the prisoner had caught hold of her feet, she would at once have realised that something abnormal was going to occur, unless you think that her head was forced under water, in which case there would be marks. There was no sign of a struggle. If you tried to drown a kitten it would scratch you, and do you think a woman would not scratch? The woman would realise the felonious intention of the man, and unless she was drugged, of which there was not a particle of evidence – would try to save herself by putting out her arms.

'There is not,' argued Marshall Hall, 'sufficient evidence on which you can safely come to an affirmative verdict that the prisoner is guilty.' There is, he said, reasonable doubt.

The judge's summing-up followed. Like Marshall Hall, he set his opinions in the context of the war. 'While this wholesale destruction of life is going on,' he said, 'for some days all the apparatus of justice in England has been considering whether the prosecution are right in saying that one man should die. And it is quite right that it should be so.' It was important, he said, to carry on 'business as usual . . . And so we, you and I, approach just as if this were a time of peace instead of one of the greatest world disturbances ever known in the history of the world, the question of whether the prosecution have proved to your satisfaction that George Joseph Smith is guilty of murder.'

More mundanely, he told the jury that they would have with

them, in the jury room, all three baths, which they were to make use of to test the theories of how the women might have drowned in them. And, in the course of his instruction, he threw in a new idea. Imagine, he said, this possibility:

> Wife to husband, 'I am going to have a bath'; husband to wife, 'All right, I will go and turn on the water for you'; husband to bathroom and turns on the water and waits; the wife comes in her dressing gown or night gown . . . The newly-married husband stays in the room, strips her, or she strips herself: 'I'll put you in the bath my dear'; picks her up – an eight-stone woman; a nine-stone woman; lowers her into the bath, but holds the knees up. There is no evidence of it; there is no evidence about pulling the knees; there is no evidence about pulling the legs . . . Consider the possibilities.

And, he told the jury, if on looking at the baths another theory occurs to you better than those which have been suggested, you are quite entitled to consider it. Also, if they could not decide exactly how the death was caused, they might still be satisfied that 'it was caused by a designed act of the prisoner'.

He reminded the jury that they were considering the death of Bessie, and that the circumstances of the other two deaths were relevant only in that context. Then, over several hours, he once again went through the sequence of events from George marrying Caroline Thornhill in 1898 to the death of Margaret Lofty in 1914. He told the jury to consider carefully the position of Bessie's body in the bath, adding: 'I do not think a doctor has any special qualification for telling you how people take a bath.' But Bernard Spilsbury's evidence, he said, was useful in pointing out the matters that the jury should bear in mind, particularly in regard to the possibility of drowning from various standing, kneeling, sitting or lying positions. 'You have heard Dr Spilsbury's evidence,' he said, 'and you must consider it.' Most crucial was the position of the legs, and also the question of the soap – which according to Spilsbury indicated 'a sudden death on immersion'.

He referred too to the evidence of Carrie Rapley, who said that George had come to her office after Bessie's death and said 'Was it not a jolly good job I got her to make a will?' 'Why do you think this was said?' asked the judge; '. . . is it the mistake that a clever man sometimes makes . . . or is it merely an incongruous remark of an unbalanced character saying a stupid thing?'

At this point George shouted out from the dock: 'You may as well hang me the way you are going on!' The judge continued, but George interrupted again, with: 'Get on, hang me at once and be done with it.' The judge resumed, but George called out again: 'You can go on for ever; you cannot make me into a murderer; I have done no murder.'

And so he went on, interrupting every few minutes with '. . . It is a disgrace to a Christian country this is. I am not a murderer, though I may be a bit peculiar.' And then again: 'You are telling the jury I murdered the woman!'

Drawing to the end of his marathon summing-up, the judge asked the jury to consider thirteen coincidences in circumstances of the three deaths, which were very similar to the coincidences that Archie Bodkin had set out. The jury must decide, he said, whether these coincidences pointed to 'a designed death and not an accidental one.'

The jury took just twenty-two minutes to find George Joseph Smith guilty of the murder of Bessie Annie Constance Mundy. The clerk of the court turned to George and said: 'Have you anything to say for yourself why the Court should not give you judgement according to the law?' He replied: 'I can only say I am not guilty.'

'Judges sometimes use this occasion to warn the public against the repetition of such crimes,' said Mr Justice Scrutton:

they sometimes use such occasions to exhort the prisoner to repentance. I propose to take neither of those courses. I do not

believe there is another man in England who needs to be
warned against the commission of such a crime, and I think that
exhortation to repentance would be wasted on you. The sentence of the Court upon you is that you be hanged by the neck
until you be dead, and that it is further ordered that judgement
be carried into execution in His Majesty's prison at Maidstone,
and that your body be afterwards buried within the precincts in
which you shall have been last confined after conviction . . .
may the Lord have mercy on your soul.

Finally, he added, 'I think this conviction, a thoroughly right
one, in my opinion, is largely due to the care and assiduity with
which Inspector Neil has pursued the threads of this complicated
case, and I have pleasure in saying so in public.' To which the
jury replied, 'Hear, hear.'

George turned to his barrister and said, 'I thank you Mr
Marshall Hall, for what you have done. I have great confidence
– great confidence – in you. I shall bear up.'

II

Dispatches

'I T IS A Sunday afternoon', wrote George Orwell in his essay 'Decline of the English Murder',

> the wife is already asleep in the armchair, and the children have been sent out for a nice long walk. You put your feet up on the sofa, settle your spectacles on your nose, and open the *News of the World*. Roast beef and Yorkshire, or roast pork and apple sauce, followed up by a suet pudding and driven home, as it were, by a cup of mahogany-brown tea, have put you in just the right mood. Your pipe is drawing sweetly, the sofa cushions are soft underneath you, the fire is well alight, the air is warm and stagnant. In these blissful circumstances, what is it that you want to read about? Naturally, about a murder.

Orwell was 12 years old at the time of George Smith's trial, and at school in Eastbourne in Sussex. When he wrote about it, thirty years later, it was as one of a handful of murders 'which have given the greatest amount of pleasure to the British public'. The cases of Crippen and Seddon were others. These crimes were products of 'our great period in murder, our Elizabethan period, so to speak', which ran between roughly 1850 and 1925, and when Orwell wrote about them they were familiar to 'almost everyone'. They were distinguished by being stories on a domestic scale, with an element of scheming and planning, and their characters looked like ordinary people living on ordinary streets. The boarding-houses of Blackpool, Southsea, Weymouth and

Weston-super-Mare were run by good working people and patronized by the middling classes. They were highly suited to this type of murder, and it was fitting that the descriptions of them in court were of stairwells, carpets, sculleries and bathrooms. And the evidence was of everyday happenings – drips of water running down a kitchen wall, the sounds of splashing, a knock at the door and bread and butter for tea.

Part of the fascination with George Smith was that he had killed his wives to gain such small amounts of money, and had invested his proceeds so conservatively – purchasing annuities. His monstrous ego and ruthlessness were fascinating aspects of his story, but so were his small mind, his petty nature and boundless capacity for self-delusion. Edgar Wallace's description of George at his trial makes the point. He is dressed, he writes,

> with a sort of suburban smartness, [he] waits alert, resentful, but wholly satisfied with his own innocence . . . He had his moments of agitation, but it was not the agitation of horror. He was angry at small inaccuracies. It pained him to hear 'I will' when he really said 'I shall'. You feel that it is vital to him that when he went out to buy potatoes his act should not be misrepresented and that it should not be suggested that he bought fish.

The central relationships of the George Smith story were as commonplace as the individuals. It was, after all, a twisted version of the everyday story of boy meets girl; and an extension of the experience, known in every family, of a young woman settling for a husband who is far from ideal, because marriage, for her, is essential. A century earlier Jane Austen had written about Charlotte Lucas, who, because she had no money and had reached the age of 27, married the ludicrous Mr Collins. At the beginning of the twentieth century, Charlotte Lucases were everywhere, and George preyed on them. A torrent of romantic words and hints of an exciting new life in Canada did the trick, not just with Bessie, Alice and Margaret, but also with Caroline Thornhill, Edith Pegler, Sarah Falkner, Flora Walters, Alice Reavil and doubtless others too.

In this golden age of murder, the newspaper reporters played their part, producing accounts of criminal trials that were written with drama in mind, highlighting those episodes 'that no novelist would dare make up', such as George playing 'Nearer My God to Thee' on the organ while Margaret lay, only a room away, drowned in the bath. They revelled in vivid descriptions. On the final day of the trial, the *Daily Express* wrote that George

> heard the sentence on him without flinching, without the flicker of an eyelid . . . his deep-set grey eyes casting a look of wicked defiance . . . His pale face was as hard and unemotional as it was on the first day. His white handkerchief peeped out of the breast pocket of his green-brown Norfolk jacket. He had given his light brown moustache an extra curl.

Somehow, the extra curl is the most telling detail – whether it was real, or imagined by the journalist.

According to the *Weekly Dispatch*, as the judge said the words 'you will hang by the neck until you are dead',

> the man clutching the dock rails flinches ever so imperceptibly, but beyond that awful, livid look on his face and the beads of perspiration on his forehead he is callous and brazen to the end. No sign of repentance, no pitiful thought for her sent young and unseeing to the grave, only that bloodless death-mask of a face, and those little cunning eyes blinking in the July light. He goes to the gallows as he has lived – brazenly.

George Smith now became prisoner no. 404 at Maidstone prison. His appeal was held on 29 July. Edward Marshall Hall argued that Mr Justice Scrutton had been wrong to admit evidence relating to the deaths of Alice and Margaret, since the Crown had established no prima-facie case for the murder of

Bessie. He said that the judge had also been wrong to allow Bernard Spilsbury and William Willcox to answer the question 'would the death of any of these women be consistent with accident?' That, he said, was for the jury to decide, not an expert witness. It was wrong, he added, for the judge to have suggested to the jury his own theory about the deaths, which was entirely unsupported by the evidence. But the appeal was dismissed, allowing the *Weekly Dispatch* another day of lurid coverage. Under the heading 'How He Heard His Doom', it wrote that George 'clutched the dock rail in front of him for a moment. But his head remained erect and he showed less emotion than many of the well-dressed women who looked down from the gallery at him and who had worked themselves up into a state of great excitement as the argument proceeded.'

While he awaited his execution, George spent much of his time with the prison chaplain, Joseph Stott. And, just as he had convinced his wives and girlfriends that he was a sincere suitor, he now persuaded the Revd Stott that he was innocent of murder. He was repentant for all his many sins, he said, but murder was not one of them. We know nothing of the character of Joseph Stott. Was he perhaps as gullible as Bessie? Or as anxious as Margaret was to see good in a man? Or was it the utter conviction that George Smith seemed to have – his ability to persuade himself that black was white, and that he was a victim not a perpetrator? When the Bishop of Croydon turned up at Maidstone to see George and to hear his confession, he too was won over, and became convinced of his innocence.

On 12 August 1915, the day before he was to be executed, George wrote to the bishop, and showed himself to be as adept in the expression of religious sentiment as he had once been in the language of romance:

I have just attended the Holy Communion, and everything now is in the hands of God, which has made me feel quite happy, inasmuch, through my perfect belief that Christ my Saviour, in whom I believe has heard my humble prayers and has accepted my true penitence and contrite heart for all my sins and has forgiven me. He now waits to receive me . . . I swear before Almighty God, who is my Judge, also to the whole world that I am innocent of the crimes for which I am convicted; thus an innocent man goes to his untimely end. Will you my Lord Bishop grant my humble request by making this my last statement known throughout the whole world.

He also wrote to his solicitor, Walter Davies, thanking him and declaring his innocence. He remained true, he said, to 'Miss Pegler, for whom my love is immortal . . . No one knows better than myself how womanly, how honourable, how lovable, noble and Christianlike she is. I have willed all my earthly goods to her [he had none]. My soul I render to my creator.' His remaining time on this earth, he said, would be passed 'in deep prayer and meditation'.

His final letter was to Edith:

Dear love,
Your pure heart and conscience free from stain helps me to believe that, whilst memory holds a seat within your sacred brow you will remember me. You are the last person in the world to whom I shall write, inasmuch as this is my last letter. I could write volumes of pathos prompted by the cruel position wherein I am now placed.

But I have too much respect and love for your feelings to do so. I have not asked for a reprieve, nor made a petition, and do not intend doing so. Since we have failed to obtain justice from the earthly judges, I prefer death rather than imprisonment. So an innocent man goes to his untimely end, a victim of cruel fate. God alone is my Judge and the King of kings. It was He who gave me a life, who ordained our coming together. My property I give to you. Don't be alone on the last day, when I shall have left this weary ark behind, where perjury, malice, spite, vindictiveness, prejudice, and all other earthly ills will have done its best, and can harm me know more. My time is occupied in solemn and deep meditation. I am preparing my soul for Him to receive. I return to the teaching which I received from my mother . . . I have gone to God with all my sins with true repentance, and asked His forgiveness and mercy on my soul. I truly believe and feel that my faithful and sincere prayers have been answered . . . I shall have an extraordinary peace, perfect peace. May an old age, serene and bright, and as lovely as a Lapland night, lead thee to thy grave. Now, my true love, good-bye until we meet again.

    Yours, with immortal love,

    George

Both letters were published in the *News of the World* that Sunday, with an account of his execution on Friday, 13 August. 'Smith walked feebly between a couple of warders, and quickly reached the drop which is only thirty or forty yards from his cell. The doomed man had to pass a portion of the open prison yard, into which the brilliant sunshine of a glorious summer morning was pouring.' Joseph Stott led the way, reciting the service for the dead. George, who was allowed to wear his own (unpaid for) clothes to his execution, remained silent.

> He must have heard on his way to the scaffold the hubbub of the large crowd which had gathered outside the prison walls. A number of well-dressed women were among the crowd, and at the windows of the cottages on the other side of the road women's heads could be seen by the score. The greater part of the male assemblage was made up of men in khaki.

The executioner, John Ellis, had arrived at Maidstone gaol the evening before. He had inspected the trap-doors in the death-shed, taken note of George's height and weight and calculated the drop required on the scaffold, and had observed George while he was in the exercise ground, hoping to get a good look at his neck. He wrote later that George's appearance had changed dramatically in prison. At his appeal his hair had been brushed and his moustache waxed, now his hair was long, unkempt and had turned almost white. 'His face was drawn and haggard, and even his moustache drooped sadly and seemed to be changing colour. His back was bent and he looked altogether like an old man.'

At a minute and a half before eight in the morning, Ellis arrived at George's cell.

I pushed open the cell door and entered. Smith was standing with his back to me, and his hands clasped behind his back. He flinched slightly as I gripped his left wrist and put the pinioning strap over it, but he made no attempt to struggle, or even to move at all. I then fastened this wrist and the other together behind his back. Having loosened his shirt neck I departed from the cell, leaving Smith in the charge of my assistant, and made with all speed for the scaffold.

The procession came forth behind me from the prison, and I stood awaiting it at the place of execution thirty yards distant. Many of those present were perhaps inclined to forget the man's awful crimes as he walked at a fair pace to his doom. But this compassion must have vanished when he presently showed that, despite the imminence of death, he was as impenitent as ever. He was facing me hardly a couple of inches off the trapdoors when he halted and exclaimed: 'I am innocent of this crime!' . . . I pulled him on to the chalk mark on the trapdoors and put the white cap over his head. While I was fixing the rope round he spoke again. 'I am innocent!' he lied once more. His last chance for righting himself with God was gone. I pulled the lever, and 46 seconds after leaving his cell Smith, the Brides Bath Murderer, was dead.

George Smith was left hanging for a full hour, as was required by law. Then Inspector Arthur Neil, who had witnessed the execution, made the formal identification of the body.

Afterwards the Bishop of Croydon wrote to Edward Marshall Hall. In prison, he wrote, George Smith was a completely changed man. 'He was softened, penitent and a convinced believer in the Christian faith . . . He asserted, with the tears coursing down his cheeks, that he had not had anything to do with the murder of these three women. He left a statement to this effect in his cell; and the last words he spoke, just as he was about to be executed were "I am innocent." I cannot, with a long experience of penitents, believe that he was not sincere in his declaration.' If George had killed his wives, then 'he must have been mad, for I am absolutely convinced that he believed himself innocent of this crime'.

Edward Marshall Hall made it clear to the bishop that, though he had defended George Smith to the best of his ability in the hope of saving him from 'the extreme penalty of the law', he was certain that he had killed his wives.

> That he did not drown them in any of the ways suggested by the evidence, or the *ex parte* suggestions of the judge, I am convinced; but I am equally convinced that it was brought about by hypnotic suggestion. I had a long interview with Smith, under very favourable circumstances, and I was convinced that he was a hypnotist. Once I accept this theory, and the whole thing, including the unbolted doors, is to my mind satisfactorily explained.

The implication of the letter was that George had hypnotized the susceptible Bishop of Croydon.

The general opinion, though, was that George Smith was not a hypnotist – but simply a particularly evil man who bullied his wives into obeying his every command. It was unfortunate that this monster had happened upon an ingenious way of drowning women without attracting attention. Maybe, in the privacy of 80 High Street, Herne Bay, the ease and speed with which he killed Bessie, and the readiness of the inquest jury to assume an accident, had given him the confidence to repeat the act in a boarding-house, with people close by. The theory, devised by Bernard Spilsbury and Inspector Neil, of the pulling up of the legs, became established in the public mind as George's method. And the certainty with which Spilsbury had answered questions in the courtroom, together with the authority that he exuded, made it seem that the legs, the 'goose skin' and the soap, were a vital part of the case, and that science had played its role in securing justice.

12

Aftermath

THE BRIDES IN the Bath case elevated Bernard Spilsbury from promising expert witness to star performer, and 'Spilsbury Called In' soon became a familiar newspaper headline, signifying that an absorbing murder mystery was to follow. His testimony at the trial of George Joseph Smith was seen as clever and brilliantly articulated; and his science – the new forensics – was regarded as fascinating, not least because it expanded the world of 'clues' in the real-life detective story. The scar on the body in Dr Crippen's cellar had, five years earlier, commanded attention worldwide. Now, the 'goose skin' on Bessie's thigh and the Castille soap that she clutched in her hand were similarly vivid images, satisfying in their own right, but all the more intriguing because they could be interpreted only by the extraordinary skills of an expert.

After the Brides' trial, Spilsbury's career took off. A string of high-profile trials allowed him to showcase qualities that were loved by the police, prosecution lawyers and juries. He always turned up at court looking magnificent; he spoke with great authority and perfect timing; his answers were clear and he presented himself as totally certain of his ground. His commonly used expressions: 'I have no doubt' and 'that is my definite opinion' seemed to sweep aside any alternative explanations. And when he added 'others may take a different view', or 'that is the most modern view' – it was clear that a community of less scientific men might not agree, but that his opinion was in every way superior. And he quickly perfected a sense of drama – an appreciation of the impact that a well-placed silence, or lowered voice, or moment of thought could have on a jury. 'Yes I appreciate that', he would say to a defence counsel offering an alternative view to his own, 'I suppose it might happen in certain circumstances.' Then, he would pause for effect, before adding, 'But it didn't happen *here*.'

In 1917 he made the news when he examined the chopped-up body parts of a French woman, Emilienne Gerard. Her head had been reduced to a pulp by repeated blows and yet, said Spilsbury, these wounds had not killed her. In fact, she had been subsequently strangled with a towel and then dismembered and decapitated by a butcher, using a butcher's knife. His reconstruction of events was specific and damning, and supported other evidence in the case. Emilienne's lover, a butcher by the name of Louis Voisin, was sentenced to hang. Spilsbury's testimony was also instrumental in the conviction of Voisin's accomplice, Berthe Roche, who went mad and died before her prison sentence was completed. Emilienne's head wounds, said Spilsbury, had definitely been inflicted by a woman – and the only woman in the frame was Berthe.

In 1922 Herbert Rowse Armstrong, a solicitor in Hay-on-Wye, was accused of poisoning his wife Kate, who had died ten months earlier. It was said that Armstrong had also attempted to kill his neighbour, Oswald Martin, by inviting him to tea and offering scones that were laced with arsenic. Bernard Spilsbury told the court in the plainest of terms that when he had examined Kate Armstrong's exhumed body he found arsenic in her intestines and her liver. Taking everything together, he said, he was convinced that she had been given a large poisonous dose of arsenic within the twenty-four hours before her death, in addition to several other huge doses in the preceding days. The judge, in his summing-up, regarded Spilsbury's evidence as factual rather than opinion, and reminded the jury that 'He is not merely theorizing.' Armstrong was found guilty, and hanged. Early in 1923, Spilsbury received his knighthood.

It is hard now to appreciate the heights to which his reputation soared, because we have no equivalent. Judges, in directing juries, gave his evidence grave significance. And, when expert witnesses were produced for the defence, they seemed to have little effect. After a trial of 1925 a medico-legal expert wrote anonymously to an evening paper: 'For some reason or other, Sir Bernard Spilsbury has now arrived at a position where his utterances in the witness box commonly receive unquestioning acceptance from judge, counsel and jury. He can do no wrong.' And by the 1930s it was rumoured that he had quipped: 'I have never claimed to be God – just his locum on his weekends off.' So great was his personal influence in his profession that he has been showered with flattering epithets. He is 'the father of modern forensics', 'the obvious prototype of the doctor-detective of modern fiction' and 'the real-life Sherlock Holmes'. The Holmes analogy was regularly tagged to him in life, and when he died, appeared in obituaries.

As time went on, though, it became obvious that a gap existed between the power of Bernard Spilsbury to influence a criminal trial and the quality of the science on offer. One man convicted of murder and about to be hanged, declared himself to be 'a martyr to Spilsburyism'. And the forensic evidence in the Brides in the Bath case does not stand up well in the cruel light of twenty-first century expert opinion. His assertion that Bessie's 'goose skin' was a sure sign of 'a very sudden death' went unchallenged in 1915, but it is now regarded as so much nonsense. In life, 'goose skin' – its medical name is cutisanisera – might be produced due to cold or to fear; but it would disappear in death. There is, though, a condition of the skin that can result from the decomposition of the body that is very similar in appearance to 'goose skin'. This is surely what Spilsbury found when he examined Bessie's body after it had been in the ground for two and a half years. Spilsbury's opinion was, as he often said himself, based on his own experience. Perhaps he had seen 'goose skin' before on the bodies of those who had met a violent death. But correlation and causation are not, of course, the same. And personal experience is not the same as a scientific sample.

The clutching of the soap is more interesting. Modern scientists would recognize what Spilsbury described as 'instantaneous death stiffening' as cadaveric spasm, a sort of 'instant rigor mortis' that can take effect when muscles are gripping, or working quite hard at the moment of death. Spilsbury's answers at the Old Bailey, though, go beyond this. In court he made it clear that, in his opinion, the soap in the hand meant not simply that Bessie had been violently gripping the soap in the moments before her death, but that she had definitely been murdered. Of course, it was the likely, common-sense, conclusion. But there is no consensus on whether such matters (in legal terms 'the ultimate issue') are best left to the expert or the jury.

Then there is the theory of the pulling-up of the legs, sending the head under the water so fast that consciousness is lost immediately and death comes suddenly. Modern science would point to the phenomenon of 'vagal inhibition' – a clear relative of the notion of 'inhibition' described by the police surgeon F. G. Crookshank in his lecture to the Medico-Legal Society in 1909. Pressure put on the vagus nerve in the neck – for instance by water rushing down the throat – can cause a rapid slowing down of the heart rate and an instant faint. Most people experiencing vagal inhibition, though, do not die as a result – instead they recover extremely quickly. George Smith appeared to be a strong man. It is quite possible that his victims passed out as he dragged them under the water and that, when they came to, they found George's hand on their heads keeping them submerged. But, in this case, some struggling would be likely and there is still a degree of mystery about how Bessie, Alice and Margaret died with so little thrashing about or noise. Perhaps Arthur Neil's dangerous experiment with the lady swimmer in a bath provided the best clue to what happened. But, without repeating it, it is hard to be sure.

These days we might ask whether he really could tell from the body of Kate Armstrong, ten months dead, the specific individual doses of arsenic that she had taken, and over what period of time. And was it really possible to say that the head of Emilienne Gerard was, without doubt, smashed in by a woman and not a man? But these questions were not asked during Spilsbury's early career. Instead, his pronouncements were treated as though they came from a great height. Due deference was paid to the medical man, to the scientist, and the public was delighted by the ingeniousness of his Holmesian deductions.

Later on, though, there was some unease among his contemporaries about the aura of infallibility that had grown up around him. By the 1920s, observed the crime writer Edgar Lustgarten, 'Spilsbury had indeed done what few can hope to do; he had become a legend in his own lifetime . . . His pronouncements were invested with the force of dogma, and it was blasphemy to hint that he might conceivably be wrong.' A professional rival, Sir Sydney Smith, was among those who grew exasperated by Spilsbury's apparent acceptance of his own myth. 'His belief in himself was so strong that he would not conceive the possibility of error either in his observation or interpretation.' He was 'very brilliant and very famous, but fallible like the rest of us – and very, very obstinate'. There can be little doubt that, on occasion, Spilsbury's errors had fatal consequences.

By the time of the Second World War, Spilsbury, who was then in his sixties, was in decline. He was living apart from his wife Edith, when, in 1940, he had the first of several mild strokes. His deteriorating health made it hard to keep up with the long, hard hours of work that he was accustomed to put in, and he began to make elementary mistakes. At the same time, personal tragedies made life intolerable. His son Peter, a doctor at St Thomas's

Hospital in London, was killed in an air-raid in 1940; his sister Constance, to whom he was very close, died in 1941; then, in 1945, another of his three sons, Alan, died of tuberculosis.

One of his last acts of professional significance was his work on Operation Mincemeat, a secret plan to deceive the Germans into believing that the Allies had immediate plans to attack Sardinia and Greece, instead of their real objective – Sicily. The mission, which was subsequently made public in Ewen Montagu's book *The Man Who Never Was*, entailed leaving false invasion plans on a dead body which would be cast into the waters off the coast of Spain. The Spanish, it was correctly predicted, would find the plans and pass them to Germany. It was essential to the operation that the Spanish military and pathologists were convinced that the body was what it seemed to be – that of a young British airman – a fictional 'Major William Martin' – whose plane had crashed into the sea. The British intelligence services consulted Spilsbury, whose advice helped fool the Spanish doctor who conducted the inevitable post-mortem. The ruse was entirely successful. The Spanish passed the information to Berlin, and Hitler ordered his troops to give priority to the defence of Sardinia and the Peloponnese.

After the war, the normal day-to-day work at the post-mortem table continued. But arthritis had damaged Spilsbury's hands, and his health slowed him down so much that it now took him a week to get through the number of autopsies that he would once have completed in a day. He pushed himself hard, nonetheless, as he was anxious about money and feared that younger men would take work from him. By 1947 he was living in a hotel in Frognal, getting by as best he could. In the winter he suffered from heavy colds and bronchitis, the debilitating effects of which were compounded by insomnia.

On 17 December that year he left his hotel after breakfast and drove to the St Pancras Coroner's Court and on to Hampstead, where he conducted an autopsy. Later that day, he gave Christmas boxes to his staff, then wrote out his last post-mortem report and posted it. In the evening he went to his laboratory in Gower Street – a small room with one window overlooking a courtyard. His test-tubes, microscopes and Bunsen burners, along with cabinets full of his case-cards, were on a wooden bench and table, much of which was covered in a layer of dust – a state of affairs which a younger, healthier Bernard Spilsbury would not have tolerated. At ten past eight a colleague was passing the room and smelled gas. When he tried the door, it was locked, so he found a watchman and obtained a pass key. When the door was opened, Spilsbury was unconscious, and probably dead already. Artificial respiration was tried with no effect, and the official time of death was given as ten minutes past nine.

The obituaries were properly reverential, detailing his out-standing contribution to the world of pathology, and describing his skills in the courtroom. 'If his methods of investigation were beyond reproach, the presentation of his facts was equally admirable', reported the *British Medical Journal*. 'He was a witness after the judge's heart, giving his evidence in clear-cut fashion, never declamatory or violent in assertion, but always sure of his case and speaking with unmistakeable authority.' The pathologist Gerald Roche Lynch wrote in the *Medico-Legal Journal*:

> As one who had known him for nearly 40 years, he appeared as a genial companion, a real friend and one who was always willing to help and advise. Generosity in every aspect was one of his characteristics. He was possessed of a great sense of humour. To others, perhaps meeting him casually and thus not able to penetrate his natural reserve, he may have given a different impression and it is true to say that he was often critical of work done by others in criminal cases and might even express himself in no uncertain terms. But this was part of his make-up in that he was always searching for the truth and an accurate presentation of the facts.

Before long, though, it became clear that the nature of Bernard Spilsbury's legacy would be a matter of fierce dispute. In 1949 an account of the Brides in the Bath trial was published as a book, and reviewers were already prepared to point out weaknesses in Spilsbury's testimony. One referred to 'some extraordinary statements perpetrated even by the great Spilsbury'. The brilliance of Spilsbury's evidence, it stated, was not in dispute. 'His unique capacity for playing the detective must have been of considerable assistance to the police.' Nevertheless, his evidence regarding the 'goose skin' was peculiar, to say the least. By the early 1950s, articles in academic journals started to appear under titles such as: 'Sir Bernard Spilsbury – a great man, a great witness or a great myth?' Further criticisms in the following years amounted to 'an orgy of denigration'.

Spilsbury was, for decades, both lauded and criticized. In the early 1980s a pathologist, Michael Green, gave a speech to senior police officers called 'Is Sir Bernard Spilsbury Dead?' He said that Spilsbury's statements in the witness box were often based on insufficient material and a lack of clinical experience; and that he was 'always ready to pontificate upon clinical symptoms and signs in conditions ranging from epilepsy and psychiatry, to congestive heart failure and alcoholic liver disease'. Green cited the distinguished gynaecologist Alec Bourne, who had spoken out against Spilsbury: 'When Sir Bernard speaks as a pathologist, I respect his opinion. When he gives a view on an obstetric matter, I hold him in contempt.'

Spilsbury's bold reconstructions of the relative positions of the assailant and the deceased, says Michael Green, remind him of Agatha Christie's Hercule Poirot and would, in modern times, be laughed out of court. Back then, though, they were accepted without question. 'No other expert could stand against him', he continues. 'Dr Bronte, his bitter professional rival, remarked that "a simple newspaper report of Sir Bernard's attendance at a mortuary or a churchyard is enough to condemn an accused man to death, even before committal proceedings have begun".'

No single expert witness now has the power of a Bernard Spilsbury. But today's expert witnesses, as a group, have more influence in criminal trials than ever before – and, culturally, they are the descendants of Spilsbury – encouraged by the police and by lawyers to be clear and concise in their evidence, to present themselves well and to avoid jargon. Consequently, the role of the expert witness is still a matter of disquiet and dispute, and decades-old questions are still fiercely debated: Are juries affected too much by the bearing and authority of an expert witness? Does the opinion of the expert witness in court (no other witness is permitted to express forthright opinions) too often seem like fact? Does the expert witness have a tendency to act as a hired gun for the prosecution or defence, rather than serving the interests of the court, and of justice? Does he, on occasion, pronounce on areas outside his expertise?

Similarly, there are still concerns about the 'science' that is admissible as evidence in court. A senior doctor, it is said, liked to start his advice to new medical students with the observation '50 per cent of what you learn now will turn out to be wrong. The problem is – we don't know which 50 per cent it will be.' And there is a saying in medicine that 'today's orthodoxy is tomorrow's outdated learning'. Both observations have some truth in them – and courts are still faced with the problem of the changing nature of science and, its close relative, the need to distinguish good science from bad. Some scientific evidence is, undoubtedly, robust – for instance, that based on DNA sampling. But other witness testimony is open to the sorts of debate that have arisen around the science of detecting sexual abuse, of 'shaken baby syndrome', the incidence of cot deaths in one family and the phenomenon of 'Munchausen's by proxy'. Debates continue about the reliability of ear-print evidence, lip-reading and handwriting. Some argue that the evidence of homeopaths should be admissible in court, others want psychologists to testify on matters such as 'false-memory syndrome'.

Even the science that secured the guilty verdict against Dr Crippen is now being questioned. Dr David Foran of Michigan State University has examined the fragment of human remains that, according to Bernard Spilsbury, was from the lower part of an abdomen and included a scar – just where Cora Crippen's scar had been. After extensive DNA testing of the specimen Dr Foran has concluded that it does it not match the DNA of Cora's descendants and is in fact tissue from a male body. And yet, uncertainties remain. There were, undoubtedly, human body parts in the cellar. So, whose were they? And what about the lengths of hair that looked like Cora's? And how was it that Cora Crippen disappeared so suddenly and never reappeared? The trial was a news sensation in America as well as Britain, and nobody in either country came forward to say she was still alive. The science of 1910 had seemed to provide a conclusive explanation of events at 39 Hilldrop Crescent. And yet, a hundred years later, the Crippen case is still, it seems, an unsolved mystery.

On such subjects it is not right to lay the blame for all the defects in the system at the door of one man. Science moves on. Bernard Spilsbury had his flaws – but so too did the defence counsel who failed to challenge him properly, the judges who regarded his evidence as faultless and the deferential juries who allowed themselves to be captivated by a remarkable individual.

Acknowledgements

I am very grateful to the many people who have helped me research this book. The staff at the British Library, the National Archives, the Wellcome Library and the newspaper library at Colindale have all been of great assistance. Particular thanks go to Bev Baker at the Nottingham Galleries of Justice who looks after Bernard Spilsbury's case cards there, and to Kevin Brown, trust archivist at St Mary's, who shared his knowledge of the hospital as it was in Bernard Spilsbury's day.

I am indebted, also, to Peter Vanezis for his expert advice on forensic pathology, and to Paul Jarvis who helped me understand the role of the expert witness in criminal trials. David Foran gave helpful guidance on his examination of the forensic evidence in the Crippen case. David Birch of Herne Bay kindly shared his own research on the Brides in the Bath case.

Judith Hibbert was a brilliant researcher and her boundless knowledge of the world of true crime was invaluable. Tom Stuttaford was hugely helpful, both with research and excellent editorial advice. Lucy Kellaway was always there, for coffee and inspiration. Janine Holland was impressive at Kew. On the home front, Tania Haimon, Agnieszka Majerowicz, Molly Robins and Carol Robins made a vital contribution. And fantastic Tom McMahon was ever-tolerant, even when his mother became obsessive about murder and seaside towns.

I would like to thank Roland Philipps and Eleanor Birne at John Murray for their much-valued support. I am also grateful to

Nikki Barrow, Bernard Dive, James Spackman, Juliet Brightmore, Margaret Wallis, Geraldine Beare and Helen Hawksfield. In addition I have benefited greatly from the wise advice of my agent Natasha Fairweather.

A special heartfelt thanks goes to Peter Ayliffe, who helped in so many ways.

TopFoto: 4 above. Mirrorpix: 3, 4 below, 7, 8. Archive of the Nottingham Galleries of Justice: 6 above. Private Collections: 1, 2, 5, 6.

Notes

Chapter 1

2   more than half a million. Nicholson, *Singled Out*, p. 13.

2   'the same income or equivalent capital.' *Matrimonial Times*, February 1910.

2   'in case anything was to happen.' Ibid.

3   the current advertisers. Ibid.

4   and her jewellery. NA: MEPO 3/225B.

4   'is a grave defect in all women.' *Nursing Mirror*, 10 July 1909.

5   'latest and newest productions.' *Bristol Times and Mirror*, 7 April 1910.

5   'an enormous mushroom on a stalk.' *Bristol Times and Mirror*, 5 April 1910.

5   'books . . . and philanthropy.' *Clifton and Redland Free Press*, 26 August 1910.

6   'speaker after speaker.' Kenney, *Memories of a Militant*, p. 120.

6   'knocked his hat about.' Willmott Dobbie, *A Nest of Suffragettes in Somerset*, p. 38.

6   barrel-organ to raise funds. *Bristol Times and Mirror*, 18 April 1910.

6   by a full set of dentures. MEPO 3/225B.

7   'how perfect teeth beautify.' *Daily Mirror*, 5 April 1912.

7   '250,000 teeth have been drawn in London this month.' British Dental Association, in *Daily Mirror*, 15 December 1906.

7   on one occasion 'touched' Bessie. NA: DPP 1/43, undated letter Bessie to Herbert Mundy, DPP 1/43, undated letter Henry Williams to Bessie.

7   her 'a much better life'. Ibid.

7   unpaid bills of about £20. Ibid.

9   'forward as much money as possible at your earliest.' DPP 1/43, typed copy of Bessie's letter.

10   'when anything was put to her by me.' MEPO 3/225B, statement of Arthur Eaton.

10   with puzzling formality, 'B. Williams'. DPP 1/43, typed copy of Bessie's postcard.

10   'matters as much as possible.' MEPO 3/225B, statement of Herbert Mundy.

11   'it's my wife who's got it all.' MEPO 3/225B, statement of Maud Crabbe.

11   'let us have cash for it?' MEPO 3/225B, statement of Arthur Easton.

11   'see that she pays you.' MEPO 3/225B, statement of Maud Crabb.

11   'not be home till tomorrow.' DPP 1/43, copy of postcard from Henry Williams to Bessie.

12   'comfortable until my return.' DPP 1/43, copy of letter from Henry Williams to Mr and Mrs Crabb.

13   'throw the pieces on the road.' DPP 1/43, undated letter from Henry Williams to Bessie.

13   'I have disgraced myself for life.' DPP 1/43, undated letter from Bessie to Herbert Mundy.

13   in debt to the landlady Mrs Crabb. MEPO 3/225B, statement of George Howard Mundy, 27 February 1915.

14   how to proceed with her life. Ibid.

14   'which she may be placed.' Davis, *The Junior Woman Secretary*, p. 3.

15   need for their future marital home. MEPO 3/225B, letter from James Griffiths.

15   acquaintance of the family, Sarah Tuckett. DPP 1/43, undated letter from Bessie to Herbert Mundy.

15   'who would be easily led.' MEPO 3/225B, statement of George Howard Mundy.

15   'been kind to Bessie.' DPP 1/43, letter from Henry Williams to Mrs Tuckett, 15 March 1912.

16 'more sorry than myself for what has occurred.' DPP 1/43, letter from Henry Williams to George Howard Mundy, 18 March 1912.

16 'a true and worthy husband.' DPP 1/43, letter from Henry Williams to Herbert Mundy, 17 March 1912.

16 'Life after all is not finished yet.' DPP 1/43, letter from Henry Williams to Mrs Tuckett, 15 March 1912.

16 'I am perfectly happy.' DPP 1/43, letter from Bessie to George Howard Mundy, 18 March 1912.

17 'do let me have a line from you.' DPP 1/43, letter from Bessie to Herbert Mundy, 21 March 1912.

17 it was as her husband had stated. DPP 1/43, letter from W. B. Lillington, 15 April 1915.

17 Henry's commitment to his marriage. DPP 1/43, letter from Baker & Co. to Herbert Mundy, 14 March 1912.

17 a thoroughly bad lot. DPP 1/43, various letters.

18 made out in her married name. DPP 1/43, letter from Bessie to Herbert Mundy, 23 April 1912.

18 'all the joy of life and the search of pleasure.' *Herne Bay Press*, 1 June 1912.

19 'Nearer my God to Thee'. *Herne Bay Press*, 11 May 1912.

20 'turning somersaults and drinking milk under water.' *Herne Bay Press*, 29 June 1912.

20 with a month's rent in advance. MEPO3/225B, statement of Carrie Rapley, 19 February 1915.

21 visit as a paying guest. DPP1/43, undated letter from Bessie to Herbert Mundy.

21 as he went about the local streets. MEPO 3/225B, statement of Percy Millgate, 15 February 1915.

21 removing a broken knocker from the front door. DPP1/43, schedule of landlord's fixtures at 80 High Street.

21 'Pictures, China, Curios and Antique Furniture bought' engraved upon it. MEPO 3/225b, letter from Surrey Police, Watson, *Trial of George Joseph Smith*, p. 105.

21 they lived 'very quietly'. MEPO 3/225B, statement of Percy Millgate, 15 February 1915.

22   'she beckoned me with her hand.' MEPO 3/225B, statement of Carrie Rapley, 19 February 1915.

22   Henry paid the lawyer's fees that day. MEPO 3/225B, statement of Phillip de Vere Annersley, 19 February 1915.

23   it had to be filled and emptied manually, using buckets. MEPO 3/225, statement of Adolphus Michael Hill, 19 February 1915.

23   'She still complained of lassitude and headache.' DPP 1/43, evidence of Frank Austin French, 15 July 1912.

24   'for I love my husband.' DPP 1/43, letter from Bessie to Herbert Mundy, 12 July 1912.

24   'I then went straight for Dr French.' DPP 1/43 and MEPO 3/225B, evidence of Henry Williams, 15 July 1912.

25   she was still clasping a large bar of soap in her right hand. MEPO 3/225B evidence of Dr Frank French, 15 July 1912.

25   there was no need for a post-mortem. Ibid.

26   underpaid him by a shilling. MEPO 3/225B, statement of Alfred Apps Hogbin, 19 February 1915.

27   'Oh well I made a will all the same.' MEPO 3/225B, statement of Carrie Rapley, 19 February 1915.

27   'as he had a latch-key.' MEPO 3/225B, further statement of Ellen Millgate, 18 February 1915.

27   'he could not sleep since he lost his wife.' MEPO 3/225B, report by Sergeant J. H. Gutteridge,10 April 1915.

27   for the same price as he had paid for it − £1 17s 6d. MEPO 3/225B, statement of Adolphus Michael Hill, 19 February 1915.

28   'sufficient strength to bear this calamity.' DPP 1/43, letter from Henry Williams to Herbert Mundy, 18 July 1912.

Chapter 2

29   the 'lower regions' of St Mary's Hospital. *St Mary's Hospital Gazette*, October 1901, cited in Rose, *Lethal Witness. Sir Bernard Spilsbury, Honorary Pathologist*, p. 12.

30   needles, twine, sponges and sawdust. Box, *Post-Mortem Manual*, p. 2.

31   curves in his rickety legs. Well. PP/SPI/1.113.

31   an operation on his adenoids. Well. PP/SPI/1.114.

31   died during an abdominal operation. Well. PP/SPI/1.119.

31   26-year-old Charlotte Parr. Well. PP/SPI/1.133.

31   did not survive a routine circumcision. Well. PP/SPI/1.142.

31   52-year-old George Smith, Well. PP/SPI/1.147.

31   'She said medicine was burning her inside. Died 9.15 p.m.' Well. PP/SPI/1.111.

31   hydrochloric acid, and died within 24 hours. Well. PP/SPI/1.131.

31   George Snow, who swallowed hydrocyanic acid. Well. PP/SPI/1.135.

32   'in locked room and gas stove turned on.' Well. PP/SPI/1.136.

32   a miscarriage and several days in great pain. Well. PP/SPI/1.165.

32   after a back-street abortion Well. PP/SPI/1.146.

32   home abortion with a knitting needle. Well. PP/SPI/1.143.

32   'extreme emaciation of child.' Well. PP/SPI/1.132.

32   '"stillborn?"' Well. PP/SPI/1.121.

34   enjoyed a respect that defence witnesses did not. Jones, *Expert Witnesses, Science, Medicine and the Practice of Law*, p. 82.

35   'fifteen doctors of all grades and shapes.' Golan, *Laws of Men and Laws of Nature*, p. 160.

36   rebuilding the credibility of 'science as a witness.' Ibid., p. 164.

37   'I spent several hours examining it.' Young, *The Trial of Hawley Harvey Crippen*, pp. 47–8.

37   not far from Holloway prison. Cullen, *Crippen: The Mild Murderer*, p. 14.

38   'I was by no means sure I was not talking to a bream or a mullet.' Seymour Hicks, *Not Guilty M'Lord*, cited ibid., p. 15.

38   and to search outgoing ships. *The Times*, 15 July 1910.

38   60,000 policemen had joined the hunt. *Daily Express*, 15 July 1910.

38　a photograph of 'Crippen's favourite seat at the hotel'. *Daily Mirror*, 28 July 1910.

39　he retrieved his revolver, and put it in his pocket. Larson, *Thunderstruck*, pp. 4–5.

40　'much more exposed to the eyes of the public than if he remained on land.' quoted in Goodman, *The Crippen File*, p. 37.

40　'Will gladly print all you will say.' Cullen, *Crippen*, p. 135.

41　'faces of the angry mob.' Dew, *I Caught Crippen*, p. 58.

42　'the chain of evidence of identification.' Ibid., pp. 31–2.

43　on her lower abdomen. Young, *Trial of Crippen*, p. 62.

44　one two-hundredth of a grain. Ibid., p. 69.

44　he had bought it for 'homeopathic purposes.' Ibid., p. 75.

44　hyoscine as a homeopathic remedy. Ibid., p. 70.

44　'morphia, strychnine, cocaine and so on.' Ibid., p. 68.

44　tested by squirting it into the eye of a cat. Ibid., p. 71.

45　connected to a case of murder. Ibid., p. 70.

45　whilst Crippen was living in the house, not before. Felstead, *Sir Richard Muir*, pp. 85–6.

47　the nature of his complaint. Lycett, *Conan Doyle: The Man who Created Sherlock Holmes*, p. 52.

47　'you probably observed the face, especially the nose.' Pearson, quoted in Liebow, *Dr Bell*, p. 131.

47　'At last there was some attempt to make it exact . . .' *The Times*, 3 October 1910.

47　meticulous preparation and his grasp of detail. Rose, *Lethal Witness*, p. 25.

47　'I fear the worst.' Felstead, *Sir Richard Muir*, p. 5.

48　Cora Crippen's operation. Trial of Crippen at Old Bailey online.

50　'we went to bed in rather a temper with each other.' Young, *Trial of Crippen*, p. 88.

50　'but I still lived with her.' Ibid., p. 89.

50　'she was always finding fault with trivial things.' Ibid., p. 90.

52　'the grossest carelessness and rashness.' Ibid., p. 158.

52　entitled to walk from the court a free man. Ibid., p. 163.

52　'I still protest my innocence.' Ibid., p. 183.

52   'Words can never tell my grief.' Marjoribanks, *The Life of Sir Edward Marshall Hall*, pp. 74–5.

53   and ran away with Ethel. Ibid., p. 281.

54   'might have preferred to believe Edward Marshall Hall.' Ibid., p. 284.

Chapter 3

55   'always healthy and bright.' MEPO 3/225B, statement of Elizabeth Rose Pratt, 30 April 1915.

55   close-knit Christian household. MEPO 3/225B, Alice's letters home.

55   'and the greatest of friends.' MEPO 3/225B, statement of Annie May Pinchin, 5 May 1915.

56   'like ladies, if they saw the way.' Abel-Smith, *A History of the Nursing Profession*, p. 23.

56   'better than he himself could have imagined?' Cited ibid., p. 18.

57   'banish such as sap your energy and faith.' Burdett, *How to Become a Nurse*, 1909.

58   the gas was put out at quarter past eleven. Ibid., 1905/1909.

58   a separate bedroom for each nurse. Ibid., 1905.

58   by 1901, the number had risen to 39,184. Abel-Smith, *History of the Nursing Profession*, p. 57, Select Committee on Registration 1905, p. 102.

59   'a revelation to a somewhat phlegmatic public.' *Nursing Times*, 6 February 1909.

59   Mr Holt – a 'confirmed invalid'. MEPO 3/225B, statement of Bertram Stone, 25 February 1915.

59   'entered the hospitals only to visit, inspect or govern.' Abel-Smith, *History of the Nursing Profession*, p. 53.

59   more nurses worked in private households than in hospitals. Ibid., p. 52.

60   so was now safeguarding a full £100 for her. MEPO 3/225B, statement of Charles Burnham, 16 February 1915.

60   able to make only occasional trips home. Ibid.

60   a life-threatening inflammation of the bowel linings. DPP 1/43,
      North British and Mercantile Co. insurance form.

60   'a strong, healthy, robust girl.' MEPO 3/225B, statement of
      Bertram Stone, 25 February 1915.

61   but he wasn't, by any reckoning, ugly. MEPO 3/225B, state-
      ment of Joseph Crossley, undated; MEPO 3/225B, statement of
      Alice Crossley, undated.

61   he was renting rooms at 80 Kimberley Road, Southsea. MEPO
      3/225B, statement of Annie Page, 25 February 1915.

61   she intended to marry. MEPO 3/225B, police report, 22
      January 1915.

61   would bring only a small bag with them. DPP 1/43, letter from
      George Smith to Elizabeth Burnham, 22 October 1913.

62   'he had never done any work and did not intend to do any.'
      MEPO 3/225B, statement of Norman Burnham, 16 February
      1915.

62   'and his father was a drinking man.' MEPO 3/225B, police
      report by Superintendent N. Wootten, 21 January 1915; MEPO
      3/225B, police report, 22 January 1915; MEPO 3/225B, state-
      ment of Elizabeth Burnham, 21 April 1915.

62   with a large seal attached to its chain. MEPO 3/225B, police
      report by Superintendent N. Wootten, 21 January 1915.

62   the visitors returned to Aston Clinton. MEPO 3/225B, state-
      ment of Annie May Pinchin, 5 May 1915.

63   cut her visit short and take George Smith away. MEPO 3/225B,
      police report by Superintendent N. Wootten, 21 January 1915;
      MEPO 3/225B, statement of Charles Burnham, 16 February
      1915.

63   taking a separate rented room. MEPO 3/225B, statement of
      Annie Page, 25 February 1915.

63   didn't mention that he was Alice's intended husband. MEPO
      3/225B, statement of Charles Pleasance, 25 February 1915.

64   she and George were married at the local register office. DPP
      1/43, marriage certificate of George Smith and Alice
      Burnham.

64 'and found it quite healthy,' said the doctor. MEPO 3/225B, statement of Harold Burrows, 25 February 1915.

64 the £100 that he had been looking after for her. MEPO 3/225B, statement of Charles Burnham,16 February 1915.

65 He signed himself G. Smith. MEPO 3/225B, letter from George Smith to Charles Burnham, 11 November 1913.

65 'I hope you and mother are well Dad.' MEPO 3/225B, letter from Alice Burnham to Charles Burnham, 22 November 1913.

66 'names, position and place of abode of your parents.' DPP 1/43, letter from Horwood & James solicitors to George Smith, 22 November 1913.

66 'Your despised son-in-law, G. Smith.' MEPO 3/225B, postcard from George Smith to Charles Burnham, 24 November 1913.

66 'take extreme measures' to obtain her money. MEPO 3/225B, letter from Alice Burnham to Charles Burnham, 24 November 1913.

66 'But take my advice and be very careful.' DPP 1/43, postcard from George Smith to Charles Burnham, 27 November 1913.

66 'she turned against us after she met her husband.' MEPO 3/225B, statement of Annie Pinchin, 5 May 1915.

66 he sent off the money. MEPO 3/225B, statement of Charles Burnham, 16 February 1915.

67 'she seemed frightened to speak.' MEPO 3/225B, report of Sergeant Stewart Williams, 3 February 1915.

67 'allowing his wife to make one.' MEPO 3/225B, statement of Charles Pleasance, 25 February 1915.

68 about noon the same day, she signed it. MEPO 3/225B, statement of Charles Wayling, 26 February 1915.

68 she should rent the room out in that time. MEPO 3/225B, statement of Annie Page, 25 February 1915.

68 'but asked no questions.' MEPO 3/225B, statement of Susannah Marsden, 9 February 1915.

69 Alice appeared to be in good health, 'and was very cheerful.' MEPO 3/225B, statement of Margaret Crossley, 10 February 1915; further statement of Margaret Crossley, undated.

70   she had 'a headache and maziness, owing to a long journey.'
     MEPO 3/225B statement of George Billing, 13 February
     1915.

70   the doctor described her as 'quite cheerful'. MEPO 3/225B,
     statement of Sergeant William Greenwood, undated.

70   His fee was 3s 6d, which George paid immediately. Watson,
     Trial of George Joseph Smith, p. 166.

71   a hot bath which she would take when she got back. MEPO
     3/225B, statement of Margaret Crossley, 10 February 1915;
     MEPO 3/225B, statement of Alice Crossley, undated.

71   'With fond love from us both.' DPP 1/43, postcard or letter
     from Alice Burnham to Elizabeth Burnham, 12 December
     1913.

71   'he had done all he could for her.' MEPO 3/225B, statement of
     Elizabeth Pratt, 30 April 1915.

72   the instruction about the water. MEPO 3/225B, statement of
     Alice Crossley, undated; MEPO 3/225B, statement of Margaret
     Crossley, 10 February 1915.

72   'Do not let us say anything now.' MEPO 3/225B, statement of
     Joseph Crossley, undated; MEPO 3/225B, statement of Margaret
     Crossley, 10 February 1915.

73   'he looked so wild and agitated.' Watson, *Trial of George Joseph
     Smith*, p. 153; MEPO 3/225B, statement of Margaret Crossley,
     10 February 1915.

73   'Alice, when you have done, put the light out.' Watson, *Trial of
     George Joseph Smith*, p. 153.

73   'fetch a doctor, fetch Dr Billing, she knows him.' Ibid.,
     p. 158.

73   'I waited on the stairs.' Ibid., p. 153.

73   'the one he was supporting her with.' Ibid., pp. 165–7.

73   together George and Dr Billing lifted Alice out of the bath.
     Ibid., p. 167; MEPO 3/225B, statement of George Billing, 12
     February 1915.

74   'only a mouthful of froth and water.' DPP 1/43, George
     Billing's evidence at the inquest of Alice Smith.

74   George Smith and Robert Valiant walked together to Blackpool

police station, MEPO 3/225B statement of Robert Valiant, 7 April 1915; DPP 1/43, evidence of Robert Valiant at the inquest of Alice Smith.

74 'The Doctor examined her and pronounced life extinct.' MEPO 3/225B, statement of George Smith, 12 December 1915.

74 'very callous and in no way distressed.' MEPO 3/225B, statement of Robert Valiant, 7 April 1915.

75 'I will wire you tomorrow' MEPO 3/225B, postcard George Smith to Elizabeth Burnham, 12 December 1913.

75 'no rings on her fingers when I carried her to the bedroom.' MEPO 3/225B, statement of William Haynes, 9 February 1915.

75 'I have never seen so much hair in a bath as there was on this occasion.' MEPO 3/225B, statement of Sarah Haynes, 9 February 1915.

76 'he wanted to get away as soon as he could.' MEPO 3/225B, statement of John Hargreaves, 9 February 1915.

76 he moved in next door, with William and Sarah Haynes. MEPO 3/225B, statement of Margaret Crossley, 10 February 1915.

76 arranged to have her buried in a public grave. MEPO 3/225B, statement of Joseph Crossley, undated.

76 'No they are too common and too poor.' MEPO 3/225B, statement of Margaret Crossley, 10 February 1915.

77 asked for details to be sent on relating to Alice's childhood illnesses. MEPO 3/225B, letter from George Smith to Elizabeth Burnham, 13 December 1913.

77 'probably through being seized with a fit or a faint.' DPP 1/43, evidence from the inquest of Alice Smith; MEPO 3/225B, information for the coroner at the inquest of Alice Smith.

78 'I wish it had been the old man.' MEPO 3/225B, statement of Alice Crossley, 10 February 1915.

78 George played the piano. MEPO 3/225B, statement of Elizabeth Burnham, 21 April 1915; MEPO 3/225B, statement of Norman Burnham, 16 February 1915.

78 'I screwed her down . . .' MEPO 3/225B, statement of John Hargreaves, 9 February 1915.

79 'This was the last I ever saw or heard of him.' MEPO 3/225B, statement of Alice Crossley, 10 February 1915.

Chapter 4

81 'the bodies pierced with holes or crushed, aroused their bantering humour .' Zola, *Thérèse Raquin*, p. 73.

81 'Attempt to destroy body in fire. In doubled up position.' Well. PP/SPI/1.298.

82 working into the night. Browne and Tullett, *Bernard Spilsbury: Famous Murder Cases of the Great Pathologist*, p. 80.

83 'a revelation of manly beauty.' Marjoribanks, *Life of Sir Edward Marshall Hall*, p. 17.

83 'endowed with pre-eminent personal beauty of the most virile type.' Ibid., p. 14.

83 'I have to create an atmosphere – for that is advocacy.' Ibid., p. 13.

83 'less skilful advocate must have given up for lost.' Ibid., introduction.

83 '*You* must take this point, there's some law in it.' Ibid., p. 14.

86 'a matter of prime importance to Government?' *Strand Magazine*, December 1904.

86 pictures of incriminating prints. *Strand Magazine*, May 1905.

87 the method of identifying human blood was now 'absolutely infallible'. *Strand Magazine*, March 1910.

87 'the scientific questions in the case.' Marjoribanks, *Life of Sir Edward Marshall Hall*, p. 291.

89 'which is so often a weakness of his class.' Young, *Trial of Crippen*, p. xvi.

93 'then obviously the gastro enteritis would increase.' Ibid., pp. 108–33.

93 'disarmingly quiet, polite and equable.' *Oxford Dictionary of National Biography*.

94 a public meeting in support of a reprieve was held in Hyde Park. *The Times*, 15 April 1912.

94 'it is entirely argumentative evidence.' Browne and Tullett, *Bernard Spilsbury*, p. 69.

94 Seddon's arrogance and self-regard. Ibid., p. 68.

94 'I shot him four times.' *Daily Mirror*, 16 April 1913.

95 'a large white feather boa and muff and dainty hat with an ostrich feather.' *Daily Mirror*, 16 April 1913.

95 'we had arranged everything so happily for this evening.' *News of the World*, 8 June 1913.

95 'I was afraid she would jump out of the window.' CRIM/139/6, statement of PC William Thornett,.

96 'It was impossible for one bullet to have caused both wounds.' CRIM/139/6, statement of Bernard Spilsbury.

97 the evidence was simply too incriminating. Hastings, *The Other Mr Churchill*, p. 66.

97 more difficult to establish an innocent motive. Ibid., p. 64.

98 'a spell of sunshine breeds motor cars as it multiplies midges.' *Daily Mail*, 4 June 1913.

98 'she produced a dainty lace handkerchief to dry her tears.' *News of the World*, 8 June 1913.

98 'violently' attracted to each other. Marjoribanks, *Life of Sir Edward Marshall Hall*, p. 318.

99 Thérèse replied, 'I don't know.' *News of the World*, 13 June 1913.

99 'his case had a strong romantic interest.' Marjoribanks, *Life of Sir Edward Marshall Hall*, p. 321.

100 enjoyed taking death-defying risks. *Daily Mirror*, 16 April 1913.

100 she gave her evidence in 'a low, clear voice'. *Daily Mail*, 4 June 1913.

101 'I loved him better than anybody in the world.' *News of the World*, 8 June 1913; Marjoribanks, *Life of Sir Edward Marshall Hall*, pp. 319–20.

101 'As an actor, he was just superb.' Felstead, *Sir Richard Muir*, p. 146.

102 a man whose tragic end had a sequel at the Old Bailey. *News of the World*, 8 June 1913; Hastings, *The Other Mr Churchill*, p. 64.

102 'she laughed heartily at their remarks.' *Daily Mirror*, 4 June 1913.

Chapter 5

103 She didn't tell Elsie her secrets. MEPO 3/225B, statement of Emily Lofty, 4 February 1915; Watson, *Trial of George Joseph Smith*, p. 182.

105 and has no womanly shape to her body. *Strand Magazine*, June 1913.

105 'and be thankful for the moment.' *Strand Magazine*, February 1913.

105 who lived away from home and worked as a teacher. MEPO 3/225B, statement of Emily Lofty, 4 February 1915.

106 hadn't seen her husband since October – and it was now December. MEPO 3/225B, letter from Major Hall Dalwood, Sheffield Police, 27 February 1915.

106 They, also distraught, complied with her request. Ibid.

107 Such people were weak-kneed parasites. *Daily Express*, 21 August 1914.

107 'waiting to be given the chance to do their duty.' *Daily Mirror*, 28 August 1914.

107 'But once aroused, he fights well enough.' *Daily Mirror*, 29 August 1914.

108 'considering his women-folk', wrote Beatrix Hudson Pile. *Daily Mirror*, 28 August 1914.

108 'who have spoilt in tennis and golf their power of delicate manipulation.' *Daily Mirror*, 19 August 1914.

108 'which the hard, sinewy hands of these would cause.' *Daily Mirror*, 24 August 1914.

109 how to make bed-socks and balaclavas. *Woman's Weekly*, September 1914.

109 'God Save the King.' *Home Notes*, 29 August 1914.

109 'on special occasions such as Christmas Day.' DPP 1/43 Yorkshire Insurance Company form, 27 November 1914.

109 she called in at the solicitor's office to collect the policy. MEPO 3/225B, statement of Thomas Rayner Cooper, 23 February 1915.

110 She hadn't told them about it. Watson, *Trial of George Joseph Smith*, p. 182.

110 'Love to you both.' MEPO 3/225B, letter from Margaret Lofty, 15 December 1914.

112 'ready money is better than a reference.' MEPO 3/225B, statement of Emma Heiss, 15 February 1915.

112 they stayed in separate rooms but had their meals together. MEPO 3/225B, police report, 22 January 1915.

112 caretakers at the register office building. MEPO 3/225B, police report, 22 January 1915.

113 John Lloyd's deposit was returned to him. MEPO 3/225B statement of Adriana Lokker, 12 March 1915; MEPO 3/225B, further statement of Emma Heiss, 12 March 1915; MEPO 3/225B, statement of Sergeant Isaac Dennison, 25 March 1915.

113 After John returned with the luggage, the couple went out. MEPO 3/225B, statement of Louisa Blatch, 12 February 1915.

114 let him know the next day if she were no better. DPP 1/43 deposition of Stephen Henry Bates, 22 December 1914; MEPO 3/225B, statement of Stephen Henry Bates, 17 February 1915; MEPO 3/225B, further statement of Stephen Henry Bates, undated; Watson, *Trial of George Joseph Smith*, p. 195.

115 he left immediately for Bismarck Road. Ibid., p. 201.

115 'She appeared quite calm and collected.' MEPO 3/225B, statement of Arthur Griffith Lewis, 10 February 1915.

116 'appeared to be quite happy with her husband.' DPP 1/43, deposition of Louisa Blatch, 1 January 1915; MEPO 3/225B statement of Louisa Blatch, 12 February 1915.

116 the gas in the bathroom was not used. DPP 1/43, deposition of Louisa Blatch, 1 January 1915; MEPO 3/225B, statement of Louisa Blatch, 12 February 1915.

116 'The sigh was the last I heard.' Watson, *Trial of George Joseph Smith*, p. 185.

117 and ask if she would like them. Ibid.

117 'I took her to him last night.' Ibid., pp. 185–6; MEPO 3/225B, statement of Louisa Blatch, 12 February 1915.

118 'The plug was drawn, and the water actually running away.' Watson, *Trial of George Joseph Smith*, pp. 189–90, MEPO 3/225B, statement of Stanley Heath, 2 February 1915.

120 Frederick Beckett took Margaret's body to the Islington mortuary. MEPO 3/255, statement of Herbert Beckett, 11 February 1915; MEPO 3/225B, statement of Frederick Beckett, 11 February 1915.

120 or that she had made a will. Watson, *Trial of George Joseph Smith*, pp. 201–2.

120 'might tend her to having a fainting attack.' DPP 1/43, deposition of Stephen Bates, 22 December 1914.

122 'thank goodness that's all over.' MEPO 3/225B, statement of Louisa Blatch, 12 February 1915.

122 accidental death due to drowning. DPP 1/43 report from the inquest into the death of Margaret Lofty; MEPO 3/225B, statement of Louisa Blatch, 12 February 1915.

122 owing Miss Blatch ten shillings in rent. MEPO 3/225B, statement of Louisa Blatch, 12 February 1915.

Chapter 6

123 'But if you strike, strike hard.' Gross, *Criminal Investigation: A Practical Textbook*, p. 15.

124 'sallow complexion and thick, black moustache.' Neil, *Forty Years of Man-Hunting*, pp. 20–30.

124 referred for a gynaecological examination. Joanna Bourke, in the *Guardian*: //www.guardian.co.uk/world/2008/nov/11/first-world-war-changing-british-society.

125 'on which were the words – Suspicious Deaths.' Neil, *Forty Years of Man-Hunting*, p. 32.

126 'walks with knees slightly bent together and feet out.' MEPO

3/225B, letter from Superintendent Wootten, 3 January 1915.

126 no concern for his wife's modesty. Neil, *Forty Years of Man-Hunting*, pp. 32–3.

127 whether George Smith and John Lloyd were the same man. MEPO 3/225B, letter to the Assistant Commissioner of Police, New Scotland Yard from Chief Constable Pringle, 13 January 1915.

127 'so little was known about the parties.' MEPO 3/225B, report of Arthur Neil, 19 January 1915.

128 'does think there was a peculiarity about his legs.' Ibid.

128 the Yorkshire Insurance Company of Bristol. Ibid.

128 Margaret had taken out the policy after a visit on 24 November 1914. MEPO 3/225B, statement of J. Tanner, 21 January 1915.

128 a payment of £700 for his client, John Lloyd. MEPO 3/225B, statement of Thomas Cooper, 23 February 1915.

129 she had left an estate of only £5. MEPO 3/225B, statement of J. Tanner, 21 January 1915.

129 'assisting us as far as is compatible with his legal position.' MEPO 3/225B, report of Arthur Neil, 22 January 1915.

129 It could not be long, thought Neil, before Lloyd returned. Ibid.

130 'his daughter's life was insured after marriage.' MEPO 3/225B, report of Arthur Neil, 22 January 1915.

130 'Why, in the face of it, the thing – legally – is impossible.' Neil, *Forty Years of Man-Hunting*, p. 35.

130 'the slightest intimation that any enquiry was being made.' MEPO 3/225B, report of police superintendent, 16 August 1915.

130 'please do not be afraid to ask me.' Neil, *Forty Years of Man-Hunting*, p. 37.

130 'and their curiosity was not aroused.' MEPO 3/225B, police report of police superintendent, 16 August 1915.

131 'Lloyd would abscond.' MEPO 3/225B, report of Arthur Neil, 24 January 1915.

131 'in case he has a gun on him.' Neil, *Forty Years of Man-Hunting*, pp. 37–8.

132 'I don't know what you are talking about.' MEPO 3/225B, report of Harold Reed, February 1915.

133 bombs that could be thrown overboard. Castle, *Fire over England*, p. 43.

133 a Zeppelin hovering over the Houses of Parliament. *Daily Express*, 5 December 1914.

133 'flies against a window-pane.' *Daily Mirror*, 17 December 1914.

133 'there was no ammunition suitable for attacking Zeppelins.' *Strand Magazine*, May 1919.

133 'before the end of the year.' *Daily Express*, 14 December 1914.

133 an invasion of 200,000 men landing at different places. *Diaries and Letters of Marie Belloc Lowndes*, 1911–47, letter to her mother, 10 March 1915.

134 'as if he could hit it by throwing stones.' *Daily Express*, 20 January 1915, 21 January 1915.

134 'carrying the war to the soil of old England!' Robinson, *The Zeppelin in Combat*, p. 64.

135 forensics was hardly a priority at the Front. Rose, *Lethal Witness*, p. 43.

135 the post-mortem room at St Mary's. Browne and Tullet, *Bernard Spilsbury*, p. 51.

135 an analysis of the viscera DPP 1/43, letter from Home Office to the DPP, 23 January 1915.

135 A delay of a few days, or a week, would make no difference. DPP 1/43, letter of 29 January 1915.

136 he has been obtaining his living by victimising women.' MEPO 3/225B, reports of Inspector Cole and Inspector Neil, 2 February 1915.

137 'making a fresh start.' MEPO 3/225B, report of Arthur Neil, 5 February 1915.

137 'in an attitude of strained attention.' *Daily Express*, 3 February 1915.

137 the slippery nature of the evidence. MEPO 3/225B, report of Arthur Neil, 2 February 1915.

138 'to her resting-place.' Neil, *Forty Years of Man-Hunting*, p. 41.

Chapter 7

142 'so that I may make enquiries.' MEPO 3/225B, letter from Superintendent Heard, 6 February 1915.

143 by which he had inherited £2,579 13s 7d. MEPO 3/225B, report of Detective Inspector Cole, 10 February 1915.

144 'Wait home for letter next post.' MEPO 3/225B, statement of Alice Reavil, 22 February 1915.

145 'If you love me come soon. Charles x x x.' DPP 1/43, letter from Charles James to Alice Reavil, 22 September 1914.

145 'the whole of my life's savings.' MEPO 3/225B, statement of Alice Reavil, 22 February 1915.

146 his stated profession was baker and confectioner, hers boot-maker. DPP 1/43, marriage certificate, George Love and Caroline Thornhill.

147 so that it could be wheeled into the town. Neil, *Forty Years of Man-Hunting*, p. 45.

147 'She was a tall, well-built woman.' MEPO 3/225B, further statement of Percy Millgate, 19 February 1915.

148 the dimensions of the Herne Bay bath. NOTT, Spilsbury case-cards for Bessie Mundy.

149 'He said it was a Turner sea-scape.' MEPO 3/225B, statement of Edith Pegler, 23 February 1915.

150 selling them shortly afterwards at a loss. MEPO /225B, statement of Edith Pegler, 23 February 1915.

152 paid one premium, before giving up the idea. MEPO 3/225B, statement of Edith Pegler, 8 May 1915.

152 'not fit to have the custody of their children.' DPP 1/43, letter from Grey & Co. solicitors, 5 May 1915.

153 living with Bessie in Herne Bay. MEPO 3/225B, further statement of Edith Pegler, 20 March 1915.

154 'a bath in a bathroom to my knowledge.' MEPO 3/225B, statement of Edith Pegler, 23 February 1915.

154 'through weak hearts and fainting in a bath.' MEPO 3/225B, further statement of Edith Pegler, 20 March 1915.

156 more than a year's salary at the needlework shop. MEPO 3/225B, statement of Flora Jarvis (Walter), 26 February 1915.

157 mission to cure 'juvenile depravity'. Carpenter, *Reforming Schools for the Children of the Perishing and Dangerous Classes and for Juvenile Offender*, preface.

158 'for all the world as if they were young convicts.' Barnett, *Young Delinquents, a Study of Reformatory and Industrial Schools*, p. 87.

158 'eighteen in the Reformatories.' Ibid., p. 95.

158 often joined the army or the navy. Ibid., p. 113.

158 farm work, laundry work and baking. Certified list, 1912, 15 (the school was then re-established as Farnborough School).

159 he opened the bakery at Russell Square. MEPO 3/225B, statement of Caroline Thornhill, 11 October 1915.

160 'and have lived there ever since.' MEPO 3/225B, statement of Caroline Thornhill, 30 March 1915.

162 'he took it away with him.' MEPO 3/225B, statement of Sarah Annie Falkner, 29 April 1915.

162 necessitated calling 121 witnesses against Smith. MEPO 3/225B, report of Arthur Neil, 18 May 1915.

Chapter 8

164 'The feet were falling off.' Zola, *Thérèse Raquin*, p. 75.

165 a man convicted of drowning small children. *Fielding, Hangman's Record*, Vol. 2.

167 the importance that Crookshank attached to 'inhibition'. *Transactions of the Medico-Legal Society*, 7 (1909–10).

168 'retention of articles in the hands of shipwrecked men.' Browne and Tullett, *Bernard Spilsbury*, pp. 50–1.

170 'saw all our anxious faces bending over.' Neil, *Forty Years of Man-Hunting*, pp. 47–8.

170 'the ordinary desire to see justice done.' DPP 1/43, letter from John Lambert, 3 February 1915.

171 'no trace capable of detection by chemical analysis.' DPP 1/43, letters of F. Marchant, March 1915.

171 'under this illusion to the end.' DPP 1/43, letter from Fred Heaven, 26 June 1916.

172 politely turned down. DPP 1/43, letter from M. Ohma, 14 April 1915.

172 'their bodies and their belongings with equal abandon.' Watson, *Trial of George Joseph Smith*, pp. 49–50.

172 'little eyes that seemed to rob you of your will.' *Weekly Dispatch*, 15 August 1915.

173 His penetrating eyes were staring darkly. *Daily Mirror*, September and October 1905.

173 a 'professional bridegroom plan'. *Weekly Dispatch*, 1 August 1915.

173 should have a powerful personality. Wingfield, *Introduction to the Study of Hypnotism*, p. 35.

174 'or young lady in business.' Watson, *Trial of George Joseph Smith*, pp. 51–2.

174 'willing subordination on the part of the wife'. Ibid., Appendix.

175 rejects the uncongenial as false. Ibid., p. 35.

175 save first the women and children. Ibid., p. 45.

175 'lies at the root of the suffrage movement.' Ibid., p. 71.

176 willing to become the wives of young Canadian farmers. *Woman's Life*, 10 June 1911.

177 'and this by a woman who says her prayers three times a day.' Watson, *Trial of George Joseph Smith*, p. 47.

178 wrote her doctor Bertram Stone. Quoted ibid., p. 53.

178 painful urination and pelvic inflammatory disease. Brown, *The Pox*, pp. 8, 122.

178 'terrible peril to our Imperial race.' Ibid., p. 116.

178 a quarter of in-patients had gonorrhoea. Worboys, 'Unsexing Gonorrhoea', p. 55.

178 'the special ailments from which they suffer.' Quoted ibid., pp. 56–7.

179 'Women who gloat over the Brides' Case'. *Weekly Dispatch*, 18 April 1915.

180 'a look at Smith in the dock.' Ibid., 1 August 1915.

181 'more than ever in his professional duties.' Marjoribanks, *Life of Sir Edward Marshall Hall*, p. 323.

182 the trial opened at the Old Bailey on 22 June. HO 144/1404/273877(1–36).

Chapter 9

183 streets of Whitechapel, Shoreditch and Hoxton. Castle, *Fire over England*, pp. 59–61.

183 but Elsie died. *Daily Express, Daily Mirror*, 1–2 June.

184 'the very quintessence of frightfulness.' Barthram, The London Airship Raids of 1915.

184 'the degree of fear they hope to inspire.' *Weekly Dispatch*, 13 June 1915.

184 and one crashed, killing the pilot. Gilbert, *The First World War: A Complete History*, p. 165.

184 the ship being longer than the building. *Daily Express*, 2 June 1915.

184 and Civil Servants who were running the war. Castle, *Fire over England*, p. 55.

184 'the greatest German of the twentieth century.' Barthram, London Airship Raids.

184 'frightfulness and infanticide.' *Daily Mirror*, 2 June 1915.

185 'is often quite as great.' *Weekly Dispatch*, 13 June 1915.

185 '*your* duty is to Join the Army *To-day*.' *Daily Express*, 25 June 1915.

187 'not suitable for everybody's ears.' *Weekly Dispatch*, 20 June 1915.

187 'a man is being tried for murder.' *Weekly Dispatch*, 27 June 1915.

188 considerable athlete in his youth. *Oxford Dictionary of National Biography*.

189 'suave-voiced, calm official-mannered.' *Weekly Dispatch*, 27 June 1915.

189 'the sordid evidence that supports the case for the Crown.' Ibid.

190 'in the enjoyment of its rights . . .' HO 144/1404/273877 (1–36).

190 'repeated over and over again.' Watson, *Trial of George Joseph Smith*, p. 67.

195 'And that was your honest opinion at that time?' 'It was.' Ibid., p. 121.

197 'he said he could not sleep without a light.' Ibid., pp. 127–9.

197 annuity of about £500 the following January. Ibid., pp. 135–6.

198 and had identified it. Ibid., pp. 141–6.

198 found it to be 'quite sound'. Ibid., pp. 148–50.

199 she replied weakly. Ibid., pp. 151–7.

200 'appeared callous and in no way disturbed.' Ibid., p. 165.

201 'Yes,' answered Dr Billing, 'very odd.' Ibid., pp. 166–9.

201 he was in a position to buy another annuity. Ibid., p. 173.

202 'a bath with the door unlocked.' Ibid., p. 181.

202 'how confident the faith within him.' *Titbits*, 10 July 1915.

204 in which John Lloyd might have drowned his wife. Watson, *Trial of George Joseph Smith*, pp. 184–9.

206 'had not preceded the drowning?' 'Exactly.' Ibid., 195–9.

206 and a date – 24.12.1914. Ibid., p. 203.

Chapter 10

207 'jet black hair and alert, thoughtful eyes.' *Daily Express*, 29 June 1915.

219 'without once turning towards the man in the dock.' *Daily Express*, 30 June 1915.

220 'with his handkerchief to his eyes.' Ibid.

Chapter 11

229 'it should not be suggested that he bought fish.' *Titbits*, 10 July 1915.
231 'as the argument proceeded.' *Weekly Dispatch*, 1 August 1915.
232 'known throughout the whole world.' HO144/1404/273877(1-36).
232 'in deep prayer and meditation.' Ibid., *News of the World*, 15 August 1915.
232 'Yours, with immortal love, George.' Marjoribanks, *Life of Sir Edward Marshall Hall*, pp. 350–1.
234 'the Brides Bath murderer, was dead.' John Ellis memoirs, in *Thomson's Weekly News*, April 1924–February 1925.

Chapter 12

243 'presentation of the facts.' *Medico-Legal Journal*, 16 (1948).
244 'I hold him in contempt.' Brownlie, *Crime Investigation: Art or Science*, 23–26.
246 'tissue from a male body.' Private correspondence of the author and Dr Foran.

Bibliography

ARCHIVES

National Archive (NA), Kew

CRIM 1/154–155
CRIM 139/6
DPP Metropolitan Police, Court and Home Office files 1/43
HO 144/1404
HO 144/1405
MEPO 3/225B

Wellcome Library (Well.)

Bernard Spilsbury case-cards
PP/SPI/1

Nottingham Galleries of Justice (NOTT)

Papers of Bernard Spilsbury

NEWPAPERS AND MAGAZINES

Bristol Times and Mirror
Clifton and Redland Free Press
Daily Express
Daily Mail

Daily Mirror
Daily Telegraph
Herne Bay Press
Home Notes
Macmillan's Magazine
Matrimonial Times
News of the World
Nursing Mirror
Nursing Times
St Mary's Hospital Gazette
Strand Magazine
The Times
Titbits
Thomson's Weekly News
Weekly Dispatch
Woman's Life
Woman's Weekly

JOURNALS

British Medical Journal
The Lancet
Medico-Legal Journal
Social History of Medicine
Transactions of the Medico-Legal Society

WEBSITES

Barthram, Adrienne, The London Airship Raids of 1915, http://www.londonairshipraids1915.co.uk/

Old Bailey http://www.oldbaileyonline.org

Oxford Dictionary of National Biography http://www.oxfordnb.com

BOOKS AND ARTICLES

Abel-Smith, Brian, *A History of the Nursing Profession*, Heinemann, 1975

Armstrong, Sue, *A Matter of Life and Death: Conversations with Pathologists*, Dundee University Press, 2008

Ashenburg, Katherine, *Clean: An Unsanitised History of Washing*, Profile Books, 2008

Barnett, Mary G., *Young Delinquents, a Study of Reformatory and Industrial Schools*, Methuen, 1913

Bartley, Paula, *The Changing Role of Women, 1815–1914*, Hodder & Stoughton, 1996

Blom, Philipp, *The Vertigo Years: Change and Culture in the West, 1900–1914*, Weidenfeld & Nicolson, 2008

Box, Charles R., MD, *Post-Mortem Manual: A Handbook of Morbid Anatomy and Post-Mortem Technique*, Churchill, 1910

Booth, Martin, *The Doctor, the Detective and Arthur Conan Doyle*, Hodder & Stoughton, 1997

Bowker, A. E., *Behind the Bar*, Staples, 1947

Brown, Kevin, *The Pox. The Life and Near Death of a Very Social Disease*, Sutton, 2006

Browne, Douglas and Tullett, Tom, *Bernard Spilsbury. Famous Murder Cases of the Great Pathologist*, Granada, 1982

Burdett, Henry Charles, *How to Become a Nurse*, Scientific Press, 1905–15

Carpenter, Mary, *Reformatory Schools for the Children of the Perishing and Dangerous Classes and for Juvenile Offenders*, C. Gilpin, 1851

Castle, H. G., *Fire over England*, Secker & Warburg, 1982

Castle, Ian, *London 1914–17, The Zeppelin Menace*, Osprey, 2008

Conan Doyle, Arthur, *The Adventures of Sherlock Holmes*, ed. and intro. Richard Lancelyn Green, Oxford University Press, 1993

—— *The Return of Sherlock Holmes*, ed. and intro. Richard Lancelyn Green, Oxford University Press, 1993

Constantine-Quinn, Max, *Doctor Crippen*, Duckworth, 1935

Cullen, Tom, *Crippen: The Mild Murderer*, Penguin, 1977

Davis, Annie, *The Junior Woman Secretary*, Pitman, 1913

Dearden, Harold, *Death under the Microscope: Some Cases of Sir Bernard Spilsbury and Others*, Hutchinson, 1934

Delafield, Francis, MD LLD, *A Handbook of Pathological Anatomy and Histology*, Bailliere Tindall & Cox, 1904

Dew, Walter, *I Caught Crippen*, Blackie, 1938

Ellis, Havelock, *Studies in the Psychology of Sex*, F. A. Davis, 1910

Evans, Colin, *The Casebook of Forensic Detection*, John Wiley, 1996

—— *The Father of Forensics. The Groundbreaking Cases of Sir Bernard Spilsbury and the Beginnings of the Modern CSI.* Berkley Books, 2006

Felstead, Sidney, *Sir Richard Muir*, John Lane, 1927

Fielding, Steve, *The Hangman's Record, Vol. 2, 1900–1929*, Chancery House Press, 1995

Forbes, Rogers Thomas, *Surgeons at the Bailey: English Forensic Medicine to 1878*, Yale University Press, 1985

Gilbert, Martin, *The First World War: A Complete History*, Phoenix, 1994

Golan, Tal, *Laws of Men and Laws of Nature: The History of Expert Testimony in England and America*, Harvard University Press, 2004

Goodman, Jonathan, *The Crippen File,* Allison & Busby, 1985

Green, Dr Michael, 'Is Sir Bernard Spilsbury Dead?', *Crime Investigation, Art or Science?*, ed. Alistair R. Brownlie, Scottish Academic Press, 1984

Gross, Dr Hans, *Criminal Investigation: A Practical Textbook*, Sweet & Maxwell, 1924

Hamilton, Cicely, *Marriage as a Trade*, Women's Press, 1981

Hare, Dr Robert D., *Without Conscience. The Disturbing World of Psychopaths Among Us*, Warner, 1994

Hastings, M., *The Other Mr Churchill*, Harrap, 1963

Howard, Thomas, *On the Loss of Teeth*, pamphlet, 1857

Humphreys, Travers, *A Book of Trials*, William Heinemann, 1953

Ingleby, Holcombe, *The Zeppelin Raid in West Norfolk*, Edward Arnold, 1915

Jackson, Robert, *Coroner: The Biography of Sir Bentley Purchase*, George Harrap, 1963

Jones, Carol A., *Expert Witnesses, Science, Medicine and the Practice of Law*, Clarendon Press, 1994

Kenney, Annie, *Memories of a Militant*, Edward Arnold, 1924

La Bern, Arthur Joseph, *The Life and Death of a Ladykiller*, Frewin, 1967

Larson, Erik, *Thunderstruck*, Doubleday, 2006

Lehmann, Ernst and Mingos, Howard, *The Zeppelins: The Development of the Airship with the Story of the Zeppelin Air Raids in the World War*, Sears, 1927

Le Neve, Ethel, *Her Life Story, Told by Herself*, London, 1910

Liddington, Jill, *Rebel Girls: Their Fight for the Vote*, Virago, 2006

Liebow, Ely, *Dr Bell: Model for Sherlock Holmes*, Bowling Green University Popular Press, c. 1982

Lycett, Andrew, *Conan Doyle: The Man who Created Sherlock Holmes*, Phoenix, 2007

Lyons, Frederick J, *George Joseph Smith: The Brides in the Bath Case*, Duckworth, 1935

Marjoribanks, Edward, *The Life of Sir Edward Marshall Hall*, Cedric Chivers, 1972

Neil, Arthur Fowler, *Forty Years of Man-Hunting*, Jarrolds, 1932

Nicholson, Virginia, *Singled Out*, Penguin, 2008

Normanton, Helena (ed.), *The Trial of Norman Thorne*, Geoffrey Bles, 1929

Pankhurst, Christabel, *The Great Scourge and How to End It*, E. Pankhurst, 1913

Parry, Leonard (ed.), *The Trial of Thomas Smethurst*, William Hodge, 1931

Peel, Dorothy, *How We Lived Then – 1914–1918 – A Sketch of Social and Domestic Life in England During the War*, John Lane, 1929

Randall, Leslie, *The Famous Cases of Sir Bernard Spilsbury*, Nicholson & Watson, 1936

Rentoul, Robert, *Proposed Sterilisation of Certain Mental and Physical Degenerates*, Edinburgh: Walter Scott Publishing, 1903

Robinson, Douglas H., *The Zeppelin in Combat*, Foulis, 1971

Rose, Andrew, *Lethal Witness. Sir Bernard Spilsbury, Honorary Pathologist*, Sutton, 2007

Sims, G. R. *The Bluebeard of the Bath: A Story of Marriage and Murder*, Pearson, 1915

Smith, David James, *Supper with the Crippens*, Orion, 2005

Symons, Julian, *Bloody Murder: From the Detective Story to the Crime Novel*, Penguin, 1985

Thomas, Ronald, *Detective Fiction and the Rise of Forensic Science*, Cambridge University Press, 1999

Thorwald, Jurgen, *Dead Men Tell Tales*, Thames & Hudson, 1966

Walton, John K., *The Blackpool Landlady: A Social History*, Manchester University Press, 1978

—— *The English Seaside Resort: A Social History 1750–1914*, Leicester University Press, 1983

Walvin, James, *Beside the Seaside: A Social History of the Popular Seaside Holiday*, Penguin, 1978

Watson, Eric, R., *Trial of George Joseph Smith*, William Hodge, 1949

Willcox, P. W. A., *The Detective Physician*, Heinemann, 1970

Willmott, Dobbie, B.M., *A Nest of Suffragettes in Somerset*, Batheaston Society, 1979

Wilson, Colin, *Written in Blood: A History of Forensic Detection*, Grafton Books, 1990

Wingfield, H. E., *An Introduction to the Study of Hypnotism, Experimental and Therapeutic*, Baillière, Tindall & Cox, 1910.

Worboys, Michael, 'Unsexing Gonorrhoea: Bacteriologists, Gynaecologists and Suffragists in Britain, 1860–1920', *Social History of Medicine*, 17.1: 41–59

Wyatt, R. J., *Death from the Skies, the Zeppelin Raids over Norfolk, 19 January 1915*, Gliddon Books, 1990

Young, Filson (ed.), *The Trial of Hawley Harvey Crippen*, William Hodge, 1920

—— *The Trial of the Seddons*, William Hodge, 1914

Zola, Emile, *Thérèse Raquin*, trans. Philip Downs, Heinemann, 1955

Index

Index